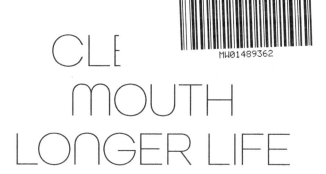

CLEAN MOUTH LONGER LIFE

What Mainstream Medicine and Conventional Dentistry Don't Know or Won't Tell You

Lina Garcia, DMD, DDS

Disclaimer

This book is intended to be an information resource only. There is no intent that this book be used for any diagnostic or treatment purposes. A specific physician/patient or dentist/patient relationship is necessary before any medical or dental therapies are initiated. In no manner should this book, or any of the information in this book, be used as a substitute for diagnosis and treatment by a qualified medical and/ or dental healthcare professional.

This book is dedicated to

My Parents and my Son
They have always inspired and
encouraged me.

Jim Marlowe
The healthiest human being on planet
earth. Jim is a true nutritional warrior and
I am extraordinarily blessed to know him.
Jim walks his talk one hundred percent
of the time. After more than twenty-five
years of collaboration, I can say with
total conviction that the world is a better
place because of Jim.

– Dr. Lina Garcia

ACKNOWLEDGMENTS

After a long journey to bring this book to completion, I am honored to thank the people who helped make it a reality.

David Nicol your unconditional support and commitment was clear in every step while editing the 2nd edition of this book. Your curiosity, intelligence, persistence, and willingness to dive in allowed you to simplify complicated facts and details. It has been a pleasure to work with you.

Dr. Joseph Grasso - shared his experience and knowledge as an outstanding osteopathic physician and partner.

Jay Hall - JJ your friendship and support is unconditional. Your ability to connect loose ends is unstoppable. Thanks for spending hours making this project possible and making my life better.

FOREWORD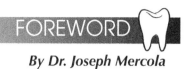

By Dr. Joseph Mercola

Congratulations on your decision to educate yourself about how your mouth influences your health. Although it might seem obvious to you that the health of your mouth influences your overall health, this is not taught in conventional medicine. When one goes to medical school, very little attention is paid to the importance of your dental health.

There is a lack of appreciation of the enormous influence that oral health and hygiene have on your overall health. Unfortunately, there is a similar ignorance regarding the importance of eating high-quality foods to achieve optimal health.

That's why I congratulate you for reading this book by Dr. Lina Garcia, a holistic dentist, whom I see for my own dental care. While the Internet is a great resource and can jump-start your learning curve, ultimately it is helpful to have a few good resources that put all the information together in one place as Dr. Garcia has done with this book.

Holistic dentists are also known as biological or environmental dentists, and they operate according to the belief system that your teeth are an integral part of your body and hence your overall health. Holistic dentists recognize that your oral health can have a major influence on other disease processes in your body. The primary aim of holistic dentistry is to resolve your dental problems while working in harmony with the rest of your body.

As a patient of Dr. Garcia for more than 10 years, I know she uses the most advanced technology to provide safe and high-quality dental care.

After treating thousands of patients for over 30 years, I am firmly convinced that if you have an optimized diet prenatally and into adulthood, you can virtually eliminate the risk of dental diseases that could otherwise lead you to see a dentist or even an orthodontist. Your body was designed to stay healthy as long as you provide it with the nutrients you need and avoid toxic influences. Dental disease is typically the result of not having these optimal exposures.

Tragically, this is not conventional wisdom, and very few families in the U.S. understand how to implement this process. As a result, nearly all of us are handicapped by poor diets we had when we were young that led to significant dental disease requiring the use of restorative interventions. I am no stranger to this process, as I had over a dozen "silver" fillings by the time I was in college. (In reality, "silver" fillings, or dental amalgams, are made of 50 percent mercury, with little to no silver at all.)

In the early '90s, I learned of the danger of "silver" fillings from watching a 60 Minutes segment with Mike Wallace. This was new information to me at the time, but once I became aware of the danger I immediately sought out my local dentist to remove the dangerous mercury fillings. I had him replace many of my silver fillings with gold crowns. This was an expensive and time-consuming intervention and little did I know at the time, my well-intentioned efforts would cause me more harm than good.

You see, I didn't understand that most dentists in the early '90s were completely ignorant about the dangers of mercury. They were unaware of the risks associated with the fact that it is a potent brain poison that can cause serious kidney damage. So when they removed mercury-amalgam fillings, they took no precautions to prevent the mercury from being dumped from the filling into the patient. This is precisely what happened to me, and as a result I suffered kidney damage that I still struggle with today, more than 20 years later.

Thankfully, the scenario is a bit better today, as about 50 percent of dentists in the U.S. are mercury-free. However, only an estimated 10 percent of these dentists fully understand the health risks associated with "silver" fillings, or dental amalgam. If your dentist is in the 90 percent that doesn't fully understand the risks associated with removing and replacing "silver" fillings, you could risk acute toxicity from mercury that is released during the removal process.

A local holistic physician, the late Dr. Tom Stone, taught me the importance of paying careful attention to oral health matters and the proper ways to do it. He educated me on the dangers of root canals and how they could devastate your health.

I seek to share this information on my website, mercola.com, to educate people on some of the risks associated with traditional dentistry. There is no question that prevention is the best strategy. Ideally, parents can implement the nutritional principles I advocate on my site and avoid fillings, root canals or braces.

So the practical challenge is how to stay current on these important dental issues. The best way to do that is to find a dentist who is trained in the principles of holistic dentistry, and reading Dr. Garcia's book is a good place to start.

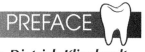

PREFACE

By Dr. Dietrich Klinghardt

As a doctor who has specialized in biological medicine for almost 40 years, I'm convinced that chronic illness is the result of a system overwhelmed by stress.

Biological Medicine acknowledges that we are part of and in interaction with the earth and everything that lives. Our bodies have evolved over several million years as robust systems with excellent self and adaptive capabilities. However, these precious skills have developed by interacting with the natural environment- whole foods, clean air, clear blue skies and natural clouds, natural periods of famine and feast, cold and warm, wet and dry, safety and fear, happiness and grief.

All of that has changed.

The microbes in our gut have to interact with artificially grown and genetically modified crops, chemical pesticides, fertilizers and herbicides, food colorings and other factors. Our air is filled with aerosols containing aluminum, barium, fluoride and other toxic substances. Our drinking water contains residues of farming chemicals, pharmaceuticals, microbes and metals. The natural geomagnetic patterns in which we have evolved have been bulldozed-over by microwave radiation from cell phone broadcasting, radar and many other sources. Our bodies get predominantly artificial input, not the needed one from nature. The damage from all sources is cumulative.

So what do our teeth have to do with this? The potential stresses to our biological system stemming from the teeth and jaw are enormous and hugely contribute to the overall toxic and stress burden. Their contribution can be up to 50% of the entire cumulative stress in any given individual. Simply this: Improperly treated dental problems play a huge role in adding to the stress on our bodies. Most dental issues can be addressed in a rational and humanistic manner, but that is not what young dentists are learning in dental school.

With the growing influence of special interests financing the universities and their dependence on the funding, the evolving science has been ignored, pushed to the side and is not translated into how things are done. The FDA still regulates mercury amalgam fillings as a device, not as something that is actually inside the body and interacts in potentially negative ways with virtually every body system ever looked at.

Fortunately, times are beginning to change. Dr. Lina Garcia has never put a toxic mercury amalgam filling in a patient and was ahead of the learning curve by decades before coming to the U.S. from Brazil. She has been a close friend and teacher to me and many others, and the holistic dentist to many of my clients, most of whom were suffering from chronic, seemingly intractable illness. She has helped my patients live better lives from the moment they met her. Lina has not only been able to solve their problems in the most gentle way but she is also one of the most gifted healers I have ever met.

Conventional dentists learn in school never to place dissimilar metals in the same mouth because they can cause galvanic corrosion. But in the same week, the same student may have to place a gold crown next to a mercury amalgam filling, violating the same rule he or she just learned. This way, students are forced to either quit or give up thinking rationally.

That's not the kind of dentistry that's practiced in the office of Lina Garcia, who had the good fortune – or made the wise choice – to study under Dr. Olympio Pinto in Brazil, one of the outstanding scientific minds in this field.

This book should be read by everyone interested in his or her own health, and I will recommend it to all my patients. The health of any nation will improve if holistic dentistry, as defined in this book, becomes the way forward in its dental schools. And it is not too late for that.

Dietrich Klinghardt, M.D., Ph.D.

CONTENTS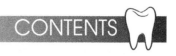

The Need to Make Well-Informed Choices

We make choices every day. Some are easy to make; others require serious deliberation. Sometimes the positive, negative, or mixed consequences are quickly apparent. On the other hand, the impact of some choices is often unknown for years. Unlike which shirt or blouse to wear, decisions about our health are critical, and we want to make wise decisions to avoid regrets.

We'd all like to think we make good decisions – ones based on careful consideration of all the relevant information, but social scientists tell us that the vast majority of them are made with our emotions rather than with our powers of reason. The tendency to make emotional decisions can be costly in health. And the danger is multiplied when there is a total lack of good information or a mass of misinformation clouds the issues.

Sometimes Critical Choices are Made for You

Add to this a situation when we are not even given a choice but are directed to follow the same path that has been worn deeply by countless others. For example, do you have a "silver" filling in your mouth? If you do, did you choose to have this filling after you and your dentist discussed other restoration possibilities, or was that choice made entirely by your dentist? If you decided to allow a "silver" filling to be placed into a tooth after considering other restoration possibilities, then at least you made a choice.

Might you have made a different choice if your dentist had told you that over half of the "silver" filling he was about to plant in your mouth consisted of mercury? Yes, these fillings contain high amounts of the same mercury the EPA calls hazardous. The EPA requires that this substance only be handled by people in full hazmat suits to avoid exposure to the vapor it emits – even from a broken fluorescent light bulb. But it's okay in your mouth? Never, not with any manipulation of the data. It is highly toxic and is tied to severe neurological disorders and other chronic diseases.

So why are dentists allowed to use mercury amalgam fillings? It may have something to do with the organization that held patents on this material: The American Dental Association. To make a truly wise choice, we first need to be well-informed, and being well-informed about "silver" fillings begins with knowing that to allow a "silver" filling containing mercury to be placed into any of your teeth could result in anything from subtle to severe consequences for your long-term health.

In Chapter 5, I will explain why using this highly toxic element in dental restorations should be viewed as an archaic practice and why you should not allow any dental material containing mercury to be placed into any of your teeth or the teeth of your children. If you already have mercury in your teeth, I will help you understand what you can do about it.

Many other choices regarding your health are made for you, often without and disclosure that there are alternative, more healthful options. Most Americans have fluoride added to their tap water under the ruse that this procedure prevents dental caries (tooth decay). If public water is already fluoridated, it is likely you did not make this choice, but you can choose alternative water sources or filter it out. Chapter 12 provides significant reasons for avoiding fluoridated water – information you do not hear in the media.

The argument that fluoride is good for your teeth is questionable at best, but the evidence of its poisonous impact on the rest of the body is not. There are reasons why most cities choose to add this toxin to their drinking water, but any propaganda that claims it is suitable for health is bogus.

I am confident you would not drink fluoridated water once you have all the data. Drinking fluoridated water because you believe it suits your teeth is a prime example of making an unhealthy choice based on misinformation or incomplete information.

Sometimes You are Unaware of a Need to Choose

We are exposed to toxins in our food, water, and air daily. Most of these exposures occur without conscious decisions. Several of these will be addressed in this book. People who are presented with all the pertinent information regarding health decisions are likelier to make the best choices for themselves. Throughout this book, you will be given the data – risks, benefits, and studies, especially regarding dental procedures and materials, that will allow you to make good decisions.

In the same way as traditional medicine, conventional dentistry is locked into specific care methods and seldom presents alternatives. Filling or extracting teeth, bridges, crowns, root canals, and implants are provided within narrow constraints based more on ease, immediate patient comfort, and appearance rather than on long-term health.

Most of these procedures have been practiced the same way by conventional dentists for decades. But just because a procedure has been around for a long time does not mean it is a practice without serious risks.

Holistic physicians refer patients to me, and holistic-minded patients (on their initiative) come to my office to have their root-canal teeth extracted because these patients have developed a degenerative disease of "unknown etiology (causes)," or they have experienced a specific symptom such as pain or a general decline in their health-related to having had a root-canal procedure. It is easy to understand how this could be true when you know that a dead, chronically infected, toxic tooth, which is what a root-canal-treated tooth is, can be a causative or aggravating factor in numerous chronic health problems.

Decisions Made for Your Dental Care Affect Your Entire Body

Even if a root canal seems to resolve a specific dental problem, I am unwilling to perform the procedure, knowing what I do about the potential consequences. It goes against my respect for the principle of "first, do no harm." Because I understand that dental procedures and materials can impact our overall health, I am committed to conservative treatments knowing that the body can resolve many issues when given the opportunity. And I don't want to treat any dental problem in such a way that produces adverse consequences in other parts of the body.

In this regard, any serious medical condition should always consider a possible connection to a person's dental history. In countless situations, I have witnessed the resolution of officially diagnosed medical conditions with the removal of "silver" fillings or the extraction and removal of the chronic infection surrounding a root-canal-treated tooth. Unfortunately, it is doubtful that a conventional physician will ever consider your dental history as part of his diagnosis. It would be best to go to a genuinely holistic-minded physician. These practitioners will almost automatically include your dental history when considering any medical condition's cause or aggravating factors.

When choosing a healthcare practitioner or dentist, doesn't it make sense to choose one who has a holistic understanding of the human body – mind and spirit – and treats you as a whole being, not just a collection of parts? As mentioned earlier, what happens in the mouth affects the rest of the body because they are inextricably interrelated.

Over the 25 years of my dental practice, I have seen many patients experience improvements in their overall health after their mercury-amalgam fillings and root-canal-treated teeth were removed. Because of this, it is reasonable to tell you that mercury-amalgam fillings and root-canal-treated teeth can be causative or aggravating factors in numerous chronic health problems or even degenerative diseases.

It is easy to understand how this could be when you're aware that every single tooth you have is a little organ, and the same blood and lymphatic fluid that flows to and through your heart and all the other organs and systems in your body also flows to and through your teeth. In addition, a complex system of nerves connects your teeth to your brain.

So, when you see the whole picture, you understand that the teeth are affected by what is going on throughout the body, and, of course, the entire body is affected by what is going on in the teeth.

Unfortunately, we usually only learn about the teeth/whole body connection and the hidden risks of conventional dental practices once we have developed at least one chronic health problem. For most of us, it is hard to believe that age-old, standard dental procedures can damage our good health. But, decades of experience have proven the relationship between several conventional dental practices and a myriad of health conditions.

Tightly controlled and powerful dental and medical establishments want people to support their complex system and costly infrastructure, regardless of whether it reflects scientific truth or effectiveness. Notwithstanding, please allow me to be a dreamer for a moment as I imagine a world in which scientific integrity and the ethical principle of "first, do no harm" have won the day. Dentists and physicians work together to properly diagnose their patients so they can address the real causes of problems that may be insidiously rooted in a patient's teeth, gums, or jawbone.

People in the media and politicians discussing healthcare reform rarely question the dogmas and practices promoted by conventional dental and medical establishments. It is as if these were settled science, even though none are.

A Need to Question the Status Quo

Changing things for the better begins with questioning the status quo. It ultimately requires making better-informed choices so that we do not wind up supporting the dysfunctional aspects of conventional dental and medical establishments. Whenever we accept and pay for a treatment, we say, "I support this."

Most likely, when you were a child and used a forbidden word or phrase, your mother chastised you for a "dirty mouth." Although I'm not criticizing you, I don't want you to have a "dirty mouth," either. However, my definition of a "dirty mouth" is quite different.

If you have any mercury in your mouth or any other type of metal restoration, and at least one root-canal-treated tooth, or if you have persisting tooth decay and gum disease, then, in the tradition of your mother, but for very different reasons, you have a "dirty mouth."

I hope that what I offer in this book will help you understand the importance of cleaning up or, even better, preventing what I call a "dirty mouth." I also hope I can contribute to helping you choose wisely, not only for yourself but for your children.

Of course, we all want to avoid regretting a wrong choice we made or that was made for us. I aim to help you understand that you have critical decisions to make when caring for your health and even protecting your smile.

The surest path to good health is to become educated (at least in general) about the different approaches to dentistry and medicine available to you before choosing for yourself or your family. With this in mind, I encourage you to seek out and create your network of practitioners – family physician, dentist, and nutritionist, for starters – who have a holistic under-standing of health and appreciate the value of working together as a team to meet your family's healthcare needs. While finding and creating your network of these practitioners will take some time, it will be well spent.

The best way to prevent disease is to build your wellness. I'm devoted to helping people learn how dental practices can improve or damage their health. I want to help you make well-informed choices that support your body, mind, and spirit health. You have choices to make. May you choose wisely!

CHAPTER 1

More than Brushing and Flossing

Many diseases that injure and kill humans today start in and are fed by a dirty mouth. I'm not just referring to dental hygiene. This is far broader than brushing and flossing. I'm talking about dental procedures and materials that are part of modern dentistry that have demonstrable links to heart disease, cancer, arthritis, dementia, and other chronic diseases. Although this reality is not common knowledge, it is well documented. As further evidence, I have seen many of these diseases resolve after my patients' dental issues have been cleaned up. Let me explain why this is true...

Natural Teeth are Living Tissues

Many don't think about our teeth as living tissue until we encounter a severe toothache. They may seem to be nothing more than solid, bone-like structures, but they are much more than meets the eye. Each tooth has an internal system containing nerves, blood vessels, pores, soft tissues, lymphatic fluid, and microscopic canals (called canela) that keep it alive and just as much a living part of the body as your organs, your skin, and your appendages.

If left untreated, an infection in your big toe can kill you. That's because that infection doesn't stay isolated in the toe. If this member of your body becomes septic and begins to turn black, aggressive action must be taken to prevent a fatal poisoning of your entire body. As unpleasant as going through life without a big toe might seem, any other dead tissue in your body must be removed to avoid that death from spreading. That's just common sense, right?

Your teeth are just as much a part of your body as any other. They are part of the human organism, and whatever affects one member of the body has ramifications for the entire body. Whether you know it or not, an infection in a tooth, gums, or jawbone will negatively impact your health and life if not treated properly.

The Devastating Divorce

Unfortunately, several decades ago, there was a very unhealthy separation between the medical realm and dentistry. Most likely, your doctor has never considered your dental health when diagnosing or treating any health issue that caused you to seek medical attention. In like manner, your dentist has probably been reticent to provide medical advice. For the most part, teeth and gums are the dentist's domain, and everything else is in the medical realm. This unwise division of the body into separate and sovereign territories is arbitrary and dangerous.

Why are substances known to be toxic to the body considered safe for permanent placement in the mouth? Why would it be considered malpractice for a physician to allow a dead toe to remain connected to the foot while allowing a dead tooth to stay in the mouth is considered a healthy practice? Neither of these dental practices makes sense to a reasoning mind, yet most dentists and doctors don't even question them.

The Restorative Remarriage

This is a book about the remarriage of dental care with all other aspects of healthcare. The improper treatment of your teeth and gums can cause other problems in your overall health. And in turn, problems elsewhere in your body can affect your dental health. I am a doctor of medical dentistry (DMD), a doctor of dental surgery (DDS), and I practice holistic dentistry.

I have written this book to help you make informed choices about dental care. (I also have a website: https://www.lina.dentist) I offer you a close look at dentistry from a holistic perspective. Taking a holistic approach to anything means focusing on the whole system and the interdependence of all the parts involved rather than paying attention to just one part of the system.

The predominant trend in healthcare today is an intense focus on just one part of the human organism rather than the human body as a whole. More physicians are specialists than general practitioners. An anonymous quote that has been circulating and morphing for over a hundred years states that "a specialist is someone who knows more and more about less and less until he knows everything about nothing." Unfortunately, there is more truth to that statement than most specialists want to admit.

By definition, a dentist is also a specialist, so the phrase "holistic dentist" seems to be an oxymoron. But when I refer to myself as a holistic dentist, I'm simply saying I am concerned with a patient's health in all respects.

Before I continue, you must be aware that not all who call themselves "holistic dentists" are genuinely interested in a patient's overall health. That means you have to choose your dentist carefully. You should interview potential dentists, talk to other patients (if possible) and learn what you can about them before making a choice.

Although you may discover what you need to be consider when you choosing a dentist throughout the book, here is a list of some realities that a genuine holistic dentist understands:

> ✓ Teeth, gums, and jawbones are not
> just connected to the rest of our body
> anatomically; they are also bound by our
> blood, lymphatic fluid, nerves, and energy
> channels, known more commonly as
> acupuncture meridians.

✓ All dental procedures and materials can affect the whole body – not just the teeth, gums, and jawbones.

✓ When a highly toxic material, such as mercury, is put in a tooth, the whole body can be adversely affected.

✓ Having any shiny metal in the mouth can cause problems in the mouth and throughout the body.

✓ In addition to causing local symptoms, an infection in a tooth, the gums, or the jawbone can also cause symptoms in other areas of the body.

✓ A dead tooth in the mouth, such as a root canal-treated tooth, will be prone to harboring chronic infection and toxicity that can hurt the whole body.

✓ When a tooth is extracted, the tooth socket must be properly cleaned so that a chronic and dangerous infection in the jawbone, called a cavitation, does not develop.

✓ Tooth decay and periodontal disease are primarily caused by poor nutrition, drugs, and inadequate oral hygiene

✓ When teeth decay, other things go wrong in the body.

✓ Even though fluoride may reduce tooth decay in some people when applied

topically, it is toxic to the rest of the body,
which means that ingesting it can create
health problems.

✓ Antibiotics commonly used in dentistry can
weaken a patient's immune system, interfere
with proper healing and cause intestinal and
systemic yeast overgrowth.

Although understanding the points listed above is
essential for practicing dentistry in a way that promotes
overall patient health, conventional dentists are not
taught them in dental school. Most conventionally
trained physicians are equally ignorant about these
things because they are not taught in medical school.

In his comprehensive book, *Biological Medicine*,
the holistic physician Dr. Thomas Rau says: "The disruptive fields which occur most frequently in the body,
causing remote illnesses in other organs, are the teeth.
So long as these disruptive factors are not eliminated,
the physician will remain unsuccessful in many cases of
chronic disease."[1]

Ultimately, the tragic consequence of not acknowl-
edging the connection between our teeth, dental treatments, and our overall health is that no attention is given
to the real cause of – and treatment for – many chronic
health problems.

------

1. Rau, Thomas. *Biological Medicine [the Future of Natural
   Healing]*. Hoya: Semmelweis-Institut, Verl. Für Naturheilkunde,
   2011. Print.

My Motivation

So that you can better understand who I am and what motivates me, I would like to share some of my personal history with you. I grew up in a community in Brazil where people appreciated the body's natural capacity for self-healing. When someone was suffering from illness or injury, the focus was on removing obstacles to healing while supporting the body's ability for recovery. The residents of my community also knew that good health was more than just a lack of discomfort, pain, or disease. They knew that good health encompassed the whole person – body, mind, and spirit – and the unimpeded flow of life-force energy.

In this culture, where "natural" healing was emphasized, I gained an appreciation for healing the whole person. I learned that helping someone heal involves more than treating an individual part of the body and that a person should never be regarded as a collection of parts or a "disease label." Unfortunately, it has become common for people to make a disease label part of their identity. You can hear it in the language they use when people say, "I am a diabetic,"; when they refer to "my arthritis,"; or even when they describe "my cancer."

But growing up in a health-conscious community, I learned to see people with disease as people who were out of balance and whose innate healing abilities had become depleted or blocked. A person with a disease always has at least one too many obstacles in the way of their healing capabilities. Suppose you have been diagnosed with an illness. In that case, the name of the disease is just a label for a symptom or set of symptoms indicating a disturbance in your body's ability to maintain or restore homeostasis or balance. Still, you are not the disease, so don't identify yourself with it!

We all have a self-healing potential that I like to call "health." Healers have learned to synchronize with their innate healing potential. They can attune themselves to "the health" within and work with their body to encourage a return to health. While growing up in Brazil, I perceived an ability to "find the health" within myself and encourage others to "find the health" within themselves.

I also became interested in exploring tooth, gum, and jaw problems' influence on the whole body. The choice I made to practice dentistry, with holistic awareness grew from my youthful fascination with the work that dentists do, together with my concerns about how the dental procedures and materials I had been treated with could be affecting my health, as well as a curiosity about why so many people with chronic health problems weren't helped by conventional medical treatments.

In trying to support and encourage my patients' healing capabilities, I have had extensive training in hands-on osteopathy and studied nutrition. Based on my studies, I will tell you that, without a doubt, what you eat and drink every day significantly influences the health of your teeth and gums. Even more than that, we need to appreciate that good nutrition contributes to the structure and function of every cell in our bodies.

I want to ensure that my patients and readers of this book understand the importance of developing proper nutrition habits to prevent tooth decay, gum disease, and other dental problems.

When I graduated from dental school, I took an oath that, to this day, encourages me. The oath said, in part: "I will strive to advance my profession by seeking new knowledge and by re-examining the ideas and practices of the past."

I hope that the oath guides you, as well as me, on our journey toward holistic dentistry.

CHAPTER 2

Do You Have a "Dirty" Mouth?

An Unhealthy Terrain

This may be earth-shattering for germaphobes: without most bacteria, we would be unable to survive. Bacteria give us an essential connection with the physical world. For example, these vital organisms free up the necessary nutrients in our food so that our intestines can absorb them. The vast majority of germs are not pathogenic – they do not cause disease. Our entire world of plants and animals depends on symbiotic relationships with microbes. If we were to rid the world of all germs, all life on our planet would die.

When your body is healthy and functioning properly, it can easily distinguish between harmful and helpful bacteria – providing a good home for the beneficial ones while controlling and sometimes eliminating pathogenic ones. On the other hand, an unhealthy body can provide a home for opportunistic, harmful germs that infect and damage tissues. The problem isn't the pathogenic bacteria but rather the unhealthy internal environment or "terrain" that allows them to grow and infect the body.

A good gardener understands the concept of healthy terrain. A frustrating part of our world demonstrates itself as weeds growing in our garden. Sure, one could spray the weeds with weed killer. But that strategy has consequences. The spray might get on the vegetables. Without a doubt, the poison will contaminate the ground. Placing an excellent organic mulch layer around the plants is a better approach. This healthy terrain would produce healthier food and improve the garden for future plantings.

The holistic practitioner should understand this relationship between pathogens and the body's terrain, seek to eliminate those conditions that disrupt it and work to strengthen the body's powerfully effective immune system to protect against infection. Infections in the mouth, whether tooth decay (dental caries), infected teeth (periodontitis), bleeding and receding gums (gingivitis), or infections in the tissues and bone surrounding the teeth, occur when there are disruptions in terrain.

Unfortunately, conventional dentists are trained to treat the infection with little or no regard for the unhealthy conditions that enabled it. I'm not casting aspersions on the motives of conventionally-trained dentists, but a failure to address the terrain and conditions that disrupt it almost guarantees a stream of repeat visits.

Sources/Symptoms of Terrain Disruption

What happens in the mouth impacts our entire being because it is an integral part of the body. This was the theme of the Chapter 1. The corollary is also true. Anything that impacts the body, positively or negatively, has a corresponding influence on the mouth. Not only is this true of the physical aspects of the body, but the spiritual as well. There are physical and spiritual stressors, physical and spiritual promoters of health. Most of what we discuss here will specifically concern oral health, but there are corresponding impacts on overall well-being.

The categories listed below are causes or symptoms of a disruption in your oral terrain. This chapter is not intended to prescribe a treatment or diagnosis but rather to help you identify those conditions that indicate a deeper problem that needs to be addressed. Succeeding chapters will provide diagnostic and treatment options.

Foreign Materials

Any attempt to meld non-living material into living tissue must be made carefully. There is not a single structure in the human body that is not alive, including teeth and bones. The biggest terrain disrupters in this category are plastics and metals. Both classes of foreign materials are commonly used for fillings and other dental restorations. Elemental mercury, the majority component in "silver" fillings, is the most dangerous. It is so much so that I have devoted the entirety of Chapter 5 to this topic.

Plastic in composite fillings, a common alternative to mercury amalgam, is not without potential toxicity. Some of the chemicals used to make these fillings can leech out and be absorbed by the digestive system and ultimately stored in the liver and fatty tissues of the body.

Most other dental restorations – such as bridges, crowns, removable partials, and implants – are also made from metals. The problems with shiny metals in your mouth include:

They all cause some degree of toxic stress.

Two or more types of metal in the mouth cause some degree of galvanic stress because of the electrical current they produce in our mouth – this only requires two or more dissimilar metals and saliva, which acts like an electrolyte solution – and the corrosion and ablation that result from the current they produce.

✓ They can provoke allergic reactions and autoimmune dysfunction.

✓ They adversely affect the flow of energy through channels of our body known as meridians.

Due to allergic reactions and potential disruption of energy flow in the body, foreign objects, especially plastics and metals, can be a continual source of toxic exposure and stress. In other words, they contribute to a "dirty" mouth as long as they are allowed to remain. In addition, metal dental restorations that touch the gums can cause them to recede, providing pathogenic germs access to the root openings in your teeth.

Dead Tissue

One of the cruelest means of execution invented was tying a dead animal or even a dead human against the skin of the one to be executed. The microbes that decompose dead matter are pathogenic to humans when they are allowed to colonize. Over time, these pathogens would infect the one carrying the corpse around and inflict a slow death.

Similarly, a person who develops gangrene in a limb must have that limb amputated to prevent inevitable death from infection spreading throughout the body. Almost instinctively, we all know this! And yet, in the name of "saving a tooth," we allow a dead tooth to remain in the mouth. The root canal procedure aims to "kill," sterilize and keep a tooth in the mouth. This practice is also so dangerous that I have devoted all of Chapter 8 to discussing root canals and the alternatives.

Detrimental Choices

Eating the wrong foods can change the biological environment in your mouth. These changes can allow pathogenic bacteria to thrive and infect your teeth and gums. Most of us know that satisfying a sweet tooth can promote tooth decay. Smoking and chewing tobacco also have a deleterious impact. And the negative consequences of these choices can be exacerbated by a failure to follow regular dental hygiene regimens such as brushing and flossing.

Choosing to stay away from the dentist until you have a severe problem can also make problems and solutions much more invasive.

Visible Infections

Visible tooth decay (a.k.a. dental caries or a cavity), bleeding or receding gums (gingivitis), tooth pain or sensitivity, and oral lesions are proof positive of a "dirty" mouth. Often these issues prompt a visit to the dentist because they are already apparent. If such problems remain untreated, they will probably worsen, and their impact will be more widespread.

Hidden Infections

Just because you are not experiencing noticeable symptoms doesn't mean you have a clean mouth. Improperly extracted teeth, dead teeth, and even nasal sinuses can provide a home to asymptomatic focal infections. These hidden infections slowly poison your body initially, without any noticeable symptoms.

Even when these oral infections lack symptomatic expression in the mouth, they have been associated with other health problems, such as heart disease, stroke, respiratory diseases, diabetes, osteoporosis, and difficulties during pregnancy. The most common of these infections is called periodontal disease. Periodontal disease is the general label used to describe a chronic infection or inflammation of the gums and the supporting structures of the teeth. The American Academy of Periodontology seeks to educate the public about research that supports what perceptive dentists inevitably recognize: "Infections in the mouth can play havoc elsewhere in the body."

Spiritual and Emotional Issues

Our mental state and spiritual health also have much to do with our physical and dental health. Anxiety, depression, fear, bitterness, and anger change the body's biochemistry and the flow of energy needed for the optimal functioning of our natural defenses and the maintenance of normal physiology. Remember, the mouth is part of the body, and those things that affect the body also affect the mouth.

Although I will not devote much attention to the subject here, maintaining your physical and spiritual health through exercise, proper rest, sleep, meditation, and prayer will positively and restoratively impact your mouth and body. Neglect of these disciplines will produce negative consequences.

The Bottom Line

You know you have a dirty mouth when you have any of the following:

✓ Periodontitis

✓ Gingivitis

✓ Oral lesions

✓ Dental caries

✓ A dead tooth

✓ An abscessed tooth

✓ At least one root-canal-treated tooth

✓ "Silver" fillings (mercury amalgam

✓ Conventional metal dental restorations
    (bridges, crowns, and removable partials)

Whether you are aware of any of these conditions, they need attention and proper treatment. If you regularly feed your sweet tooth, smoke or chew tobacco, or don't regularly brush and floss your teeth, you likely have a "dirty" mouth. In addition, if you consider dental work in the future, you will want to avoid those dental practices that disrupt your oral terrain.

The critical thing to remember is that what goes into your mouth seldom – if ever – stays in your mouth! Eventually some of it will migrate to other parts of your body.

CHAPTER 3

What Does the State of My Mouth Indicate?

Why Holistic Dental Examination is Essential

Conventional doctors and dentists often treat the body as a collection of unrelated parts. This strategy works with machines but not with living organisms. If the starter in your car isn't working, a simple replacement of the starter will solve the problem, and you'll be on your way. When dealing with the human body, we often talk about isolated anatomical structures and systems, but all these physical parts and structures, with the mind and the spirit, function as an integrated whole. Effective treatment requires a holistic approach. Simply stated, what happens in your mind, spirit, and body impacts what occurs in your mouth and vice versa. Here are some examples of what I mean.

Contrary to popular opinion, hard brushing is not the primary cause of receding gums. Although aggressive tooth brushing is not helpful, clenching and grinding the teeth are generally the cause. This abnormal activity forces the roots to move and the gums to recede. But even these behaviors are merely symptoms of a deeper etiology. Usually, teeth grinding and clenching are an improper response to excess stress, and effective treatment must address the stress issues in tandem with treating the physical manifestation of receding gums.

Certain medications can also adversely affect gum tissues. That is why a thorough examination includes a medical history and a list of medicines you take. This leads back to the rationale for the medication. Usually, drugs are taken to provide symptomatic relief to an underlying condition that has developed because the rest of the person's being is out of balance. These can often be adequately addressed with lifestyle changes involving nutrition, exercise, proper sleep, and nurture of the mind and spirit. Unlike medications that are toxic to the body, these lifestyle adjustments nurture the body's terrain, making it much more able to function correctly and keep opportunistic forces in check.

Another holistic correlation that conventional dentistry never considers concerns the patient's blood type. Over the years, I have seen a direct link between blood type and the propensity to develop specific dental problems. More specifically, a person with Type A blood who overeats sugar will tend toward gum disease, whereas someone with Type B or O blood who overeats sugar will tend toward tooth decay. Similarly, a person whose metabolism is much more efficient at converting fats and proteins to energy than carbohydrates tends to have more gum disease when eating a low-fat, high-carbohydrate, or vegan diet. Chapters 10 and 11 provide more specifics on the importance and "how-tos" of eating in harmony with your body's metabolic tendencies.

Indeed, any dentist can treat a cavity in a tooth, but if not treated holistically, the probability of more cavities, dental infections, and ultimately dead teeth increases dramatically. These, in turn, will impact other functions in your body. Everything that happens in your body, mind, and spirit affects the whole being. Any healthcare that fails to treat the entire being can set up a cascade of health issues in the future.

The Scope of a Holistic Dental Examination

As a holistic dentist, I aim to design a treatment plan that will provide the best care for immediate problems and help them experience optimum dental (and overall) health well into the future. And since the health of the mouth is inseparably linked to the health of the body, diligence in gathering all relevant data is essential.

Most conventional dentistry fails at this point. Treating a cavity, an abscess, a broken tooth, or receding gums as isolated conditions may provide some immediate relief. Yet, it almost guarantees the manifestation of more extensive problems in the future. Just like chronic ingestion can be treated with an anti-acid, a failure to address the condition's cause means the sufferer will continue to take Tums® or pop Prilosec® until a more extensive intervention is required.

That's why I start my examination with an extensive medical history. I need to know the patient's experiences with accidents, major surgeries, antibiotics, vaccinations, medications, and previous and current medical conditions. Then, I ask about eating preferences, habits, exercise routines, and activity levels to evaluate physical and nutritional status. In addition, I like to know the patient's blood type because this helps provide important insights into their body's propensity toward certain conditions.

Since excess stress works against the body's ability to heal, I usually interview the patient to determine job type, family dynamics, and how the patient typically deals with the pressures of life. The answers to these questions help me form a picture of the patient's overall health and ability to heal.

Then, an oral exam in combination with X-rays provides a wealth of information about the dental history, overall health, and nutritional issues. If the X-rays show a high level of previous dental work, I will ask many more questions to determine possible causes for their dental conditions. The number and type of dental restorations, abnormal wearing of the teeth, and inflamed or bleeding gums are all factors that indicate problems beyond the teeth that must be addressed for long-term success. The aggregate picture from all sources will help me provide a better diagnosis and prognosis.

The diagnostic examination should include cone beam tomography when the dental history includes extractions or one or more root-canal-treated teeth. Unlike X-rays, which provide a two-dimensional image, cone beam images give a three-dimensional view. This allows the detection of cavitations (pockets of infections in the jawbone due to incomplete tooth extraction) or under or around a root-canal-treated tooth (periodontitis). Often, these infections are asymptomatic. But just because there are no symptoms – in the mouth – the toxins they pump into the bloodstream and lymphatic system can wreak havoc in organs and tissues throughout the body.

CHAPTER 4

How Should You Care For Cavities or Chipped Teeth?

The Goal

It is essential to remove any decayed tooth from your mouth. All dentists and patients agree on that fact. The real question is what should be done to restore tooth structure for future protection and to enable proper biting and chewing.

Since natural teeth are best designed for that purpose, I always want to preserve as much of any natural tooth as possible while limiting any disturbance to the mouth's natural terrain. No dental restoration is as good as our natural teeth; the more natural teeth that can be saved, the better for your mouth and your long-term health. A conservative approach that chooses a restoration that preserves as much of the healthy portion of the tooth as possible will always serve you well. This approach also limits the amount of foreign, potentially toxic material – terrain disrupters – needed to make the restoration.

There are two types of dental restorations: direct and indirect. Fillings are direct, and all others are indirect. We will discuss the advantages and disadvantages of each below.

Direct Dental Restorations

Direct restorations are called this because the repair is prepared and formed on the tooth in the mouth. These restorations are called fillings, the most commonly used restorations performed today. A filling is a direct restoration used to substitute for part of a tooth's structure. There are two types of fillings employed, and they are distinguished by the materials used:

✓ Mercury amalgam fillings ("silver")

✓ Composite fillings (white with an attempt to match the color of the tooth)

All cavities require drilling or grinding away the tooth's decay and any structurally weak areas before restoration. Additionally, fillings require some healthy tooth enamel to be removed to anchor the filling securely. After preparation is complete, a soft or malleable filling is then put into the space that has been created.

Mercury Amalgam Fillings

There is nothing to recommend this type of resto-ration and much that condemns it. The entire next chapter is devoted to discussing the health dangers asso-ciated with mercury amalgam fillings. Some dentists still use this filling type because it is easy and inexpen-sive. Cheap and easy are not good reasons to endanger the patient's or the dentist's and staff's health who must handle hazardous material.

If you already have one or more mercury amalgam fillings, there are reasons to consider replacing them. These reasons and important cautions are thoroughly covered in the next chapter.

Composite Fillings

Composite, or plastic, fillings are light-curing mate-rials, so a dentist has to shine a special light on these fillings for them to harden and set correctly. Because composite fillings are considerably more fragile than enamel, they are only appropriate for relatively small restoration needs, especially anterior (front) teeth with no occlusal (chewing) forces. When used to restore chewing surfaces, they are prone to fracture and replacement.

The advantage of composite fillings is that they closely resemble the natural tooth material and are cosmetically pleasing. They are easy to place and rela-tively inexpensive. Still, they are prone to fracture when exposed to chewing forces and can leech toxins into your mouth and body.

Composite filling materials contain plastics that contain endocrine disruptors (EDC or hormonal disruptors) one of is Bisphenol A (BPA) but there are composites that are BPA free.

Indirect Dental Restorations

Indirect restorations are prepared, formed, and hardened outside the mouth and then cemented in place. The materials used for these restorations are much more durable than filling materials. There are three basic types of indirect restorations:

✓ Crowns, caps, or veneers

✓ Inlays

✓ Onlays

Crowns (Caps)

A crown is a full-coverage restoration to cap or completely cover a tooth. In preparing a tooth for this most extensive indirect restoration, ALL of the cusps and enamel on a tooth are drilled away. Drilling a tooth down to a small stub is necessary to create a base on which the crown is placed. After this, the dentist makes an impression or three-dimensional rendering of the tooth so that the crown can be cast or milled to mimic what has been removed and to fit over the part of the tooth that remains. When the crown is ready, the dentist makes any necessary "fine-tuning" adjustments and cements it into place.

Because preparing a tooth for a crown requires the removal of **all** the tooth's enamel, whether damaged or not, this procedure weakens a tooth and jeopardizes its long-term health. A crown is needed only when much of a tooth's natural structure has already broken off or has been drilled away.

Although conventional dentists frequently recommend this procedure, you should ask why a crown would be better than a more conservative restoration like an onlay. As part of making an informed choice, tell your dentist that you want to protect as much of your natural tooth structure as possible.

When an inlay or onlay can adequately restore a tooth's integrity and function, why drill it down to a stub to put a crown on it? We need to think conservatively to avoid causing unnecessary stress to a tooth. The less a troubled tooth is drilled on, the better! The more a troubled tooth is drilled on, the more likely it is to die, and having a dead tooth in your mouth is not conducive to good health!

I have seen many new patients who brought in X-rays from other dentists. Those X-rays were taken before the other dentist placed a crown on a tooth. From my interpretation of many of these X-rays, it was clear that many teeth could have been restored with an onlay or inlay.

While I recognize that a crown is sometimes necessary, I have seldom had to use one. Dentists who consider the best treatment for the long-term health of a tooth will never recommend a crown as their first choice when an onlay or inlay can restore the integrity and function of the tooth.

Inlays and Onlays

The difference between an inlay and an onlay is the extent of the restoration. An inlay is smaller and always placed in the natural depression of a molar, surrounded by tooth structure, including the cusps (the higher chewing part of a molar). It replaces the missing inner part of a tooth just as a filling does. In contrast, an onlay is more extensive and replaces one or more cusps of a tooth. Using an onlay to restore a tooth is like giving the tooth a partial crown.

In preparing a tooth for an inlay or onlay, only the decayed, structurally weak, or fractured portion of the tooth is drilled. Healthy tooth tissue is left intact. Next, a three-dimensional rendering of the remaining tooth is created by making an impression or using digital imaging technology. The restoration is cast or milled using the rendering to mimic the tooth's missing portion. The finished restoration is then cemented into place.

Preparing a tooth for an inlay or onlay allows a dentist to follow a more conservative treatment. More specifically, an inlay or onlay involves much less drilling and cutting on the natural tooth structure than preparing a tooth for a crown requires. Because inlays and onlays replace only the compromised part of the tooth, they allow for preserving as much of the natural tooth as possible, including much of the precious enamel, the hard outer layer of a tooth, and the most protective part of its structure.

Tooth enamel is the hardest substance in the human body and rivals diamond as the hardest substance on earth. Preserving as much of the tooth as possible (and especially the enamel) helps keep it viable. The tooth will be less stressed if a dentist can save more of it. And just as importantly, preserving more of the tooth means less foreign material will be needed for the restoration. Less foreign material means less possibly toxic exposure. As both a dentist and a dental patient, I want to see as much of a tooth saved as possible.

Choosing the Right Dental Materials

After deciding how a tooth should be restored, the next decision, which can have subtle to significant effects on your long-term health, involves choosing the material that should be used in the restoration. No material is perfect, of course, but it makes sense to consider the functionality, durability, cost, appearance, and, more importantly, the impact the material may have on your overall health.

Often, in conventional dentistry, there needs to be more consideration of the impact restoration materials may have. Plastics, the main component in composite dental materials, leech toxic materials endocrine disrupting chemicals (EDCs) and hormonal disruptors. In addition, they have inferior strength, which makes them prone to breaking, especially when they are used to restore a chewing cusp.

Among the various metals used for restorations by conventional dentists, two of the most common are fillings containing mercury and crowns containing nickel. Of course, mercury is highly toxic, especially to brain cells, and nickel is known to be carcinogenic. Yet in conventional dentistry, these metal restorations are promoted as being the cheapest, most durable, and easiest to put in place. But please remember that while mercury and nickel may save a few dollars at the dentist, they can be very costly for your health!

In dental school, we are trained to tell our patients how durable an all-metal restoration is and that the only advantage of a porcelain restoration is that it looks the most like a natural tooth. Of course, aesthetics are a consideration, especially for teeth highlighted when we smile. So, if you insist on having a porcelain crown, a conventional dentist will likely recommend a porcelain-fused-to-metal restoration. This option will be justified with the argument that you'll have the strength of metal while still having a white, tooth-like appearance.

The Dark Side of Shiny Metals

Restorations that are made from elemental, shiny metals, especially mercury but also nickel and other metals, can damage our health for one or more of the following reasons:

1. Metals cause some degree of toxic stress.
2. Metals cause some degree of galvanic stress due to both the electrical current they produce in our mouth and the corrosion and ablation that result from the current.
3. Metals can provoke allergic reactions and auto-immune dysfunction.
4. Metals adversely affect the flow of energy through channels of our body known as meridians. Because our teeth are connected to the meridian system (also known as acupuncture meridians), whatever a dentist does to a tooth can affect the flow of energy through that meridian and, ultimately, affect organs or glands on the same meridian.

The Beauty of Porcelain, Ceramic, and Zirconium Dioxide (Zirconia)

The best dental materials are non-reactive (inert), non-galvanic, and exceptionally durable. These include porcelain, ceramic, and zirconia. Although using such materials requires more time, special equipment, and skill, the results are cosmetically and holistically superior. Not only are these materials superior in their strength, they readily match the color and feel of a natural tooth. More importantly, however, these substances are inert; they don't interact with or react to the tissues and saliva in the mouth. In addition, they do not conduct electricity.

CHAPTER 5

Why Are "Silver" Fillings So Dangerous?

The Problem

First, you must understand that the word silver in "silver" fillings has more to do with its silvery appearance than with the composition of the filling material. The main component of a "silver" filling is elemental mercury, which generally comprises 50 to 54 percent by weight – and other metals such as silver, copper, zinc, and others.

On its website, the Environmental Protection Agency (EPA) states that mercury is a neurotoxin – poisonous to the central nervous system, including the brain. The site goes on to declare:

Exposures to metallic mercury most often occur when metallic mercury is spilled, or when products that contain metallic mercury break, so that mercury is exposed to the air. If you are concerned about your exposure to metallic mercury, you should consult your physician.

Metallic mercury mainly causes health effects when inhaled as a vapor where it can be absorbed through the lungs. Symptoms of prolonged and/or acute exposures include:

✓ Tremors;

✓ Emotional changes (such as mood swings, irritability, nervousness, excessive shyness);

✓ Insomnia;

✓ Neuromuscular changes (such as weakness, muscle atrophy, twitching);

✓ Headaches;

✓ Disturbances in sensations;

✓ Changes in nerve responses

✓ Poor performance on tests of mental function.

Higher exposures may also cause kidney effects, respiratory failure and death.[1]

To answer the question, "Why do dentists fill teeth with a known neurotoxin and a substance that is hazardous to the environment and human health?" we must step back in history. The danger of using mercury has been known for over 200 years. In the 1800s,

---

1. https://www.epa.gov/mercury/health-effects-exposures-mercury

the American Society of Dental Surgeons required its members to pledge not to use mercury-amalgam fillings. But since mercury amalgam was so easy to use, did an adequate job of filling cavities, and was inexpensive, more and more dentists decided to use it anyway. Unfortunately, the American Society of Dental Surgeons lasted only from 1840 to 1856. The dentists who used mercury amalgam had a better business model and more customers. When they formed the American Dental Association (ADA) in 1859, they gained control over dentistry in the United States.

Today, a large (but declining) percentage of dentists still use fillings containing mercury because it is easy and less expensive. The ADA continues supporting dentists who use them.

I was in Europe teaching a group of holistic physicians how dental procedures and materials can affect the whole body. At some point, I mentioned that I would publish my book on holistic dentistry shortly. When I also said that I thought my chapter on the hazards of mercury-amalgam fillings was significant because many Americans were unaware of the danger, the news came as a surprise to the physicians, especially since six European countries – Norway, Denmark, Sweden, Ireland, Slovakia, and Finland – have either banned or are planning to ban the use of mercury in dentistry. The European Commission has published draft legislation to phase out dental amalgam in 2025.

After many years of denying that mercury leeches out of amalgam fillings, supporters of their use finally acknowledged, relatively recently and quietly, that mercury does come out of these fillings.

Mercury is the only metal in a liquid state at room temperature and vaporizes into poisonous gas. Inhalation of invisible, odorless mercury vapor is the primary source of elemental mercury poisoning. After it's inhaled, the vapor is absorbed by the lungs and enters the bloodstream. Mercury vapor is continually released from amalgam fillings, and activities such as chewing, brushing, grinding, and drinking hot beverages increase the vapor released.

Even though mercury is one of the most regulated substances in the United States, there is no limit to the number of these fillings a dentist can put into someone's teeth. The EPA has classified mercury as hazardous waste and regulates the discharge levels of elemental mercury and mercury compounds into the air, water, and landfills. The Food and Drug Administration (FDA) regulates mercury levels in food, drugs, cosmetics, and medical devices. The Occupational Safety and Health Administration (OSHA) issues regulations on mercury in the workplace and worker exposure to mercury substances. State and local governments, boards of health, and industries that use mercury can also regulate its use and any emissions it produces. Yet, no regulatory steps have been taken to reduce a dental patient's exposure to mercury from dental fillings!

Holistic physicians and dentists know from their clinical experience that chronic, low-level mercury poisoning can directly cause or contribute to many symptoms, ailments, or diseases in dental patients with mercury fillings. It can be challenging for any holistically-minded person to understand why the practice of using highly toxic mercury in dental fillings when much safer, functionally equivalent, affordable, and cosmetically pleasing restoration materials have been available for a long time.

With that in mind, all dental patients should know that when a dentist is working with a mercury-amalgam filling, and the mercury is outside of the mouth, it is considered a hazardous material. Dentists are taught not to touch mercury amalgam while preparing or packing it into a patient's tooth. Any mercury amalgam waste from dental treatments should be stored in a tightly closed container filled with an appropriate liquid to prevent mercury vapors from escaping because mercury vapors are hazardous to our health. And according to the EPA and the ADA, when disposing of dental material containing mercury, a dentist is **not** supposed to toss it in a garbage can, flush it down a drain or toilet, or dispose of it in a landfill because the mercury would create an environmental hazard.

The ADA admits, "Small amounts of mercury vapor can be released from amalgam during placement, mastication, and brushing." Still, it adds, "No correlation has been found between the small amounts of mercury released ... and any adverse health effect."

Mercury is the worst of the shiny metals used in dentistry because it is highly and directly toxic to human cells, especially brain and nerve cells. But this product is also dangerous for the same reasons that other elemental, shiny metal restorations are. As discussed in previous chapters: metals in the mouth cause some toxic stress. This occurs because all metals cause galvanic stress because of the electrical current they produce in our mouth (which requires only two or more dissimilar metals and saliva, which acts like an electrolyte solution) and the corrosion and abrasion that result from the current.

Are you suffering from mercury poisoning?

Mercury poisoning can be challenging to diagnose. The onset of symptoms varies based on your genetic makeup and individual sensitivity, so you may experience symptoms of toxicity but not make the connection between the symptoms and your mercury-amalgam fillings.

The first symptoms, resulting from some injury to brain cells and nerve cells, include tremors, anxiety, irritability, insomnia, headaches, numbness, and depression. Other symptoms include poor coordination, memory loss, tingling in the hands and feet, and abnormalities in electroencephalography (EEG) recordings, which measure brain wave activity.

After long-term exposure to low levels of mercury vapor, symptoms can include psychiatric effects, respiratory damage, cardiovascular problems, kidney damage, gastrointestinal problems, and oral disorders, such as inflammation and discoloration in the mouth's soft tissues.

When I was in dental school in the 1980s, the symptoms of mercury poisoning were never mentioned. Treating cavities with mercury-amalgam fillings was accepted as part of dental school dogma because these fillings had been around for many decades. It was unquestionably assumed to be safe, while all contrary evidence was completely ignored.

However, since elemental mercury, when used in dental work, can poison the cells in our body, the most relevant question to consider is our tolerance for mercury. Our tolerance is determined by how well our body can get rid of the mercury once it gets into us, together with our ability to repair or compensate for the cellular damage caused by the mercury. The human body's capacity for detoxifying mercury is highly variable. This is a big part of what is known as biochemical individuality, which means that people can differ anywhere from a little to a lot in the efficiency at which the biochemical processes of detoxification and the utilization of nutrients occur.

An example of this is the consumption of alcohol. Some people have a high tolerance for alcohol and can have many drinks before they show the effects of being intoxicated, while others will feel intoxicated from just one drink. This is true for any substance that is essentially toxic to the human body.

So, suppose you have mercury-amalgam fillings in your teeth. How do you know if your body is doing an excellent job of getting rid of the mercury and repairing or compensating for any cellular damage it causes?

To begin to answer this question, consider your current state of health. Suppose you are free of any symptoms caused by low-level but chronic mercury poisoning and experience relatively good health. In that case, your body is efficient at getting rid of mercury and repairing or compensating for the cellular damage it causes. However, if you are struggling with one or more of the symptoms previously listed, and especially if you have been told by a physician that he or she cannot find "anything wrong" and that it all must be "in your head," it is reasonable to consider at least the possibility that your body may be affected by mercury leeching out of your fillings.

Of course, many other factors are involved in someone's susceptibility to chronic health problems, such as genetic tendencies, diet, the level of contact with or consumption of toxic substances, and the level of stress (both physical and emotional). But shiny, elemental mercury can cause health problems, and its vapor comes out of fillings, so having mercury in your teeth can, at the very least, make it harder for you to stay healthy.

Because of biochemical differences between people, it's appropriate to acknowledge that some people don't seem to be harmed noticeably by the mercury leeching out of their amalgam fillings. But it's also fair to recognize that some people are injured, in both noticeable and unnoticeable ways, by the mercury vapor released by their amalgam fillings. It is also important to note that one's natural ability to mitigate the toxic effects of any poisonous substance is not fixed or guaranteed. As our toxic exposures, stress levels, and state of health change over time, so will our body's ability to handle these threats to health.

Your Choice

Without a doubt, no one should allow another mercury amalgam filling to be placed in the future. Good alternatives are readily available, are more cosmetically pleasing, and pose less health risk. Chapter 4 in this book provides several options for conventional dental fillings.

The actual decision involves whether you keep existing mercury amalgam fillings. Removing these fillings will be an additional expense and may or may not immediately change your health status. If unsure, research the health hazards of elemental mercury and evaluate your present state of health regarding the symptoms of mercury poisoning. If you decide to have the mercury removed from your mouth, there are other things to consider.

If the supporters of mercury-amalgam fillings had to prove with long-term studies that putting mercury into someone's mouth was free from longterm ill effects – something, by the way, that has never done – the matter would be quickly resolved, and mercury would no longer be used as a material to fill cavities. Given the current direction of conventional dentistry, I think it's unrealistic to expect a professional association promoting mercury-amalgam fillings as "safe" for the past 150-plus years to change its position. Fortunately, you don't have to wait for a professional association to change its position. You can set a new standard for good dental care in your life.

Removal of Mercury-Amalgam Fillings

If you decide to have your mercury-amalgam fillings removed – even if it's only for cosmetic reasons – caution is essential. It is critically important to find a dentist who is aware of mercury exposure's dangers and well-trained in using the equipment and procedures necessary to protect everyone present.

Unfortunately, dentists worldwide drill on mercury-amalgam fillings daily without regard for the increased exposure that can result from this procedure. Consequently, patients, as well as the dentist and dental staff, can become ill. However, when the process is done correctly, there is minimal exposure to mercury vapor. Therefore, before you decide who will do the work, find a dentist who understands and is equipped to perform the necessary procedures.

Those procedures need to include the following:

- ✓ Constant cooling of the tooth with water to prevent the release of more vapor
- ✓ Extra vacuum suction to remove vapor and particles
- ✓ Removal of the amalgam in chucks by cutting rather than by drilling or grinding
- ✓ Proper apparel and drapes to avoid skin exposure to mercury for patients and staff

✓ Appropriate coverings for the patient's eyes and nose

✓ Use of a rubber dam over the patient's tooth

✓ Respirators or masks, as well as gloves, for the staff

✓ A well-ventilated office (with cleansing house plants)

After the filling is removed, the dentist must dispose of the waste amalgam so it does not harm people or the environment. Amalgam waste cannot simply be tossed in the trash, washed down a drain, flushed down a toilet, or disposed of in a landfill. The EPA requires handling all elemental mercury as a toxic-waste disposal hazard. All amalgam particles must be placed in special, air-tight containers and taken to an approved waste carrier for recycling or disposal.

Only a dentist who understands these precautions and is equipped to remove and handle mercury this way is a dentist you want to do the work!

Nutrition and Detoxification

Following the proper nutrition guidelines is vital to helping your body recover from the effects of mercury-amalgam filling replacement. Before I remove any such fillings, I suggest nutritional guidelines to my patients that boost their immune systems and neutralize toxicity. See Chapter 10 for a thorough discussion of this critical matter.

In addition, a high-quality, nutrient-dense diet appropriate for the patient's metabolism is essential, both before and after the removal process, to support the body's ability to detoxify and eliminate mercury as efficiently as possible. I have found some foods beneficial for many of my patients. They include fresh cilantro, dried seaweed, dulse, kelp, and the green algae chlorella, as well as raw butter and fresh, raw coconut, which are sources of fresh, raw fat.

After the fillings are removed, I prescribe a homeopathic detoxification kit to help the body excrete mercury and bacterial toxins and begin to repair tissues. I also encourage my patients to engage in therapeutic sweating using a sauna. Eliminating toxins by sweating is a powerful way that our body cleanses itself.

CHAPTER 6

When Gums Are Reddened, Swollen, or Bleeding

Gums are an essential part of the oral terrain and often indicate potentially serious dental problems when they stray from a healthy appearance. Proper gum care is an integral part of oral health and the overall health of your body. A holistic approach to dental care sees all the structures in the mouth as an essential part of the body, mind, and spirit and addresses the problems associated with ailing gums with that mindset.

Disease in any part of the body is rarely limited to that part. It indicates there are most likely disturbances, deficiencies, and disruptions in the body-wide terrain (ecosystem) that allow opportunistic forces to gain a foothold. Suppose the practitioner diagnosing a dental problem fails to grasp that reality. In that case, the diagnosis will be incomplete – if not altogether wrong – and the treatment may address localized symptoms but will leave the door open for more severe problems to return or manifest elsewhere.

Other than dental caries (cavities), dentists commonly diagnose and treat two other diseases of the mouth: gingivitis and periodontitis. The significant differences between the two have to do with the severity and extent of the disease. Although both manifest in the gum tissues, the initiating causes and eventual extent of damage are not limited to these tissues. The diagnoses must extend beyond identifying and treating the disease symptoms. If healing is to be optimal, the reasons the inflammation or infection has taken hold in the first place must be discovered. Then, those causal or exacerbating factors must be addressed where possible.

Differing approaches to gum disorders

Conventional dentistry believes that bacteria in the mouth are the culprit in all gum diseases and tooth decay. That is a dangerously limited view. Let me give you a real-life analogy to demonstrate that problem with this narrow construct. Humans live in an ecosystem filled with a massively complex and diverse spectrum of organisms – many of those are microorganisms that live inside and outside our bodies and are essential for our existence on this planet.

In the same way, many species of mammals coexist in the world around us. Squirrels, raccoons, opossums, prairie dogs, foxes, bats, groundhogs, etc., share your world, depending on where you live. Each animal has a purpose and a part in maintaining an ecological balance. In other words, all these creatures are an essential part of the terrain. To regard them as adversaries because they decide to invade and occupy our yards and homes may lead us to disturb the natural balance and create an even more significant problem.

Like you, I don't want a raccoon in my home. So, how do I prevent this from happening? There are three basic options:

✓ **Nuclear Option**: Hire someone to eradicate all the raccoons within 5 miles of my house by placing poison bait throughout the neighborhood. This might keep these creatures out of my house, but it will also kill other animals and undoubtedly create a worse imbalance in the world around me.

✓ **Limited Warfare Option**: Carry a shotgun around the house and shoot any raccoon that happens to get in. Again, this would work, but shooting a gun in my home will create a nasty mess and might cause severe damage to the structure of the house and my furnishings.

✓ **The Protected Terrain Option**: Prevent a raccoon from entering my home by closing my doors, windows, and screens.

The same options are available for protecting ourselves from microbial infections:

✓ **Nuclear Option**: Disinfect our environment and our body with germicidal agents. Some folks feel that microbes are the enemy and must be eradicated wherever they might live. If these people were successful, we would all die. In her book *Allies and Enemies: How the*

World Depends on Bacteria, microbiologist
Anne Maczulak says that as long as
humans can't live without carbon, nitrogen,
protection from disease, and the ability to
digest their food thoroughly, they can't live
without bacteria.[1]

✓ **Limited Warfare Option:** Just like "shooting"
all the animal invaders that come into our
house, the administration of antibiotics
(i.e., "against life") will kill pathogens.
Unfortunately, this approach damages the
patient's internal terrain microbiome and
hinders the immune system, making another
infection more likely and dangerous.

✓ **The Protected Terrain Option:** Maintain the
terrain of the mouth and body. This strategy
keeps opportunistic microbes from taking
over without endangering the planet's health
and causing damage to our bodies. Many
means to accomplish this require closing the
windows and doors – lifestyle habits and
situations which create opportunities for
pathogens to gain a foothold. As a holistic
dentist, this is the strategy that I employ with
tremendous success.

A healthy body has all the necessary mechanisms
to keep opportunistic microbes from getting a foothold
in your mouth and the rest of your body. Unfortunately,
a treat-the-symptoms allopathic approach often hinders,

---

1. Maczulak, Anne, *Allies and Enemies: How the World Depends
   on Bacteria*, Financial Times Press, July 07, 2010.

disrupts, or blocks those mechanisms. Consequently, problems eventually worsen or develop in other parts of the body.

A holistic approach to diagnosing gum disorders

Diagnosing any health issue requires a thorough understanding of the patient. The practitioner needs to know:

✓ Lifestyle (occupational and recreational)

✓ Health habits (nutrition, exercise, and sleep),

✓ Medical history

✓ Dental history

✓ Results of comprehensive blood tests

Additionally, a dentist requires an oral exam that checks for cavities, oral lesions, structural abnormalities, loose teeth, and the patient's bite. X-rays and cone beam tomography may also be necessary. The more complete a picture the holistic practitioner has of you as a person, the better the outcome of treatment will be.

Conventional dentistry and medicine generally focus on symptom relief. Even when other factors are identified, they are poorly addressed or wholly ignored. Instead, treatment is usually limited to dental procedures, antibiotics, and pharmaceuticals that often exacerbate or cause new problems.

What is gingivitis?

Gingivitis (gingiva="gums" and itis="inflammation) is a gum infection that causes visible, inflamed gums.

This first stage of gum disease often includes bleeding when brushing or flossing, tenderness, swelling, and reddening. The symptoms may also include noticeable puss pockets on the gum tissue or between the teeth. But no lasting tissue damage or health complications generally occur if adequately treated before progressing to periodontitis.

What are the common symptoms of gum disease?

Possible Symptoms	Gingivitis	Periodontitis
Redness	Definitely	Definitely
Bleeding	Definitely	Definitely
Swelling	Definitely	Definitely
Soreness	Yes	Yes
Pockets of infection resulting in pus between teeth and gums	Likely	Likely
Pain with chewing or biting	Likely	Likely
Receding Gums	Possibly	Likely
Infected Bone	Possibly	Definitely
Distinctive foul odor	Definitely	Definitely
Loosening of the teeth – this allows the teeth to move, increases the gaps between teeth, and bite changes	Possible	Yes

What is periodontitis?

Periodontitis (peri="around" and odont="tooth" and itis="inflammation) is a severe infection of the bone around the tooth that can cause tooth movement, tooth loss, and necrosis of tissues, bones, and teeth. Although bad breath almost always accompanies gingivitis, periodontitis produces a characteristic odor due to the decomposition of bone tissue. Patients with either or both diseases often attempt to mask these odors by chewing gum, exacerbating their gum condition by increasing stomach acidity. It is very uncommon for periodontitis to present in young children – even those diagnosed with gingivitis – probably because many of the causes of this infection are seldom present in children.

A periodontal infection must be addressed as soon as it is suspected because of the progressive damage to bone and teeth. In addition, this focal infection can also travel to other areas of the body and initiate disease there.

How should gum disorders and diseases be diagnosed and treated?

Imagine a man with undiagnosed diabetes and a 3-pack-a-day smoking habit who becomes concerned that his gums bleed every time he brushes his teeth. He makes an appointment with a conventional dentist who, upon oral examination, finds very red, receding gums. "You have a case of periodontitis," he tells the patient. "We need to do a deep and thorough teeth cleaning. I need to plane some of your teeth, and I'll prescribe an antibiotic you must take faithfully. We have some time right now if you'd like." After the procedures, the man leaves the office, heads to the pharmacy, and gets his prescription, feeling like all his dental problems have been successfully addressed.

What are the common causes of periodontal disease?

Possible Causes	Likelihood
Dental Issues	
Inadequate brushing and flossing	Likely
Ill-fitting dental appliances	Likely
Maladjusted bite from tooth movement, ill-fitted dental restorations, bridges, crowns, and partials)	Likely
Digestive Disorders	
GERD	Likely
Acid reflux	Likely
Leaky gut	Likely
Unhealthy intestinal biome	Likely
Eating Disorders	Likely
Diseases	
Oral herpes	Likely
Diabetes	Definitely
Leukemia	Likely
Pernicious anemia	Likely
Thrombocytopenia	Likely
Hemophilia	Likely
HIV/AIDS	Definitely
Hormonal Imbalances	
Menopause	Definitely
Pregnancy	Definitely
Hormone therapies (replacement/supplementation)	Likely
Stress	Likely

What are the common causes of periodontal disease? (Cont.)

Possible Causes	Likelihood
Nutritional Deficiencies	
Too little animal fat in the diet – especially for people whose metabolic predisposition prefers protein/fat and those who have Type B and O blood	Likely
Vitamin C deficiency (scurvy)	Likely
Vitamin K deficiency	Likely
Other Possible Causes	
All drugs	Likely
Poor dietary choices (sugary and gummy foods)	Likely
Dry mouth	Likely
Teeth clenching and grinding (usually due to stress)	Likely
Tobacco use (smoking and chewing)	Definitely

Even if the periodontitis improves in the short term, this man is still in grave danger because of his diabetes, smoking habit, poor nutrition, and, most likely, the development of atherosclerosis. The dental procedures and antibiotics did not and will not eliminate any of these issues. At the same time, the antibiotics will cause potential flora and fauna imbalances in the mouth and the gut, further disrupting the body's terrain and making him vulnerable to additional health problems.

In contrast, a dentist who thinks holistically would know there was much more going on than periodontitis and would likely involve a nutritionist and a holistically thinking doctor to address this patient's obvious and perhaps hidden issues. Those issues may include stress, digestive problems, prescription drugs, chronic disease, poor nutrition, lack of sleep, lack of exercise, or a combination of factors. Until the root issues are addressed, the practitioner only puts a Band-Aid on potentially health-threatening and life-threatening conditions. It only makes sense that addressing the real problem is the only way to restore health.

Although a periodontal infection can cause teeth to move, to be loose, or to hurt when you bite or chew, other possible causal factors may be the real problem. Changing how your teeth come together (your bite) can be responsible for pain, even without an infection. Many factors can alter your bite, including ill-fitting dental restorations (fillings and crowns), dental appliances (partials, orthodontic braces, devices to curb snoring or address TMJ), and clenching or grinding your teeth. These factors can also provide an environment that encourages periodontal infections or other dental problems.

Dental devices and orthodontic appliances that move teeth too quickly can strangle circulation to your teeth, cause nerve damage, and even kill the affected teeth. The planned movement of teeth must be done slowly enough to avoid these consequences. If you are using a device in your mouth to stop snoring, reduce apnea, or treat TMJ and are experiencing tooth loosening, movement, or pain, an adjustment should be made, or an alternative treatment should be explored.

Necessary caution: Even though the root causes of any gum disorder generally originate beyond the mouth, a bacterial infection, when present, *must be* eradicated. This is in addition to addressing any other suspected causes of the problem. That eradication usually includes deep cleaning and tooth planing to remove the infection and the plaque in which it lives. In addition, I have successfully used ozone therapy (See Chapter 14) laser light (See Chapter 15) and carefully prepared and applied hydrogen peroxide therapy. These effectively restore a natural terrain in the mouth without the need for an antibiotic that introduces many other health risks.

CHAPTER 7

What if I have a diseased or dead tooth?

Introduction

If you have a diseased tooth that is still alive, most likely you are experiencing some degree of pain – the kind that sends you to the dentist, even if you dread sitting in a dentist's chair. On the other hand, if you have dead teeth in your mouth – this would include root-canal-treated teeth, a tooth that is undergoing internal resorption (a progressive destruction of the inside of the tooth), or an asymptomatic abscessed tooth – the infection may or may not be producing painful symptoms. In many ways, this is a much more severe condition.

Living tissues have mechanisms that protect against degeneration, which always occurs once death sets in, while dead tissues do not. In every other part of the body, when tissues are dying or dead, removal is vital to prevent a potentially lethal septic infection. People who have advanced diabetes often have their toes, feet, or part of their legs removed for this very reason.

Although the decomposition and infection in dead and dying teeth do not progress as rapidly, the pathogens and toxins generated can lead to life-threatening issues in other parts of the body. Once the inner part of the tooth becomes infected, the tooth cannot be restored; it must be extracted.

Extracting an Infected or Dead Tooth

No one wants a gaping hole in their smile where a tooth once resided. Depending on the location, even the thought of a missing tooth can be traumatic. Most conventional dentists know this and want to avoid tooth extraction if the patient is willing to undergo a root canal treatment. The dangers of root-canal-treated teeth are thoroughly discussed in the next chapter. If, in the future, you are placed in a position of having to "save" or extract an infected or dead tooth, I strongly recommend that you opt for extraction and a tooth replacement option such as a partial, a bridge, or an implant.

The Extraction

Many dentists inject the patient with an anesthetic with epinephrine to reduce the amount of bleeding. These drugs cause all your blood vessels to constrict, which increases blood pressure and reduces the overall movement of blood throughout the body. Restricting blood flow helps make the extraction process less messy and more accessible for the dentist. Still, a healthy blood flow to any wound is the body's way of bringing nutrients, antibodies, leukocytes, and phagocytes that fight infection and promote healing.

Another consideration involves the way the tooth is extracted. When an extraction is too aggressive, it tears more gum and bone tissue and increases the risk that the tooth will break during the process. It does take longer to work with the bone and gums not to rush the procedure, significantly lowering the risk of needing to fish for broken tooth fragments and a better post-operative outcome. This technique also lessens the injury, speeds healing, and reduces post-procedure pain.

But wait, there's more...

Since a dental infection almost always extends to the periodontal ligament and the jawbone, tooth extraction should involve more than pulling out the tooth. Any remaining periodontal ligament must be carefully removed, and infected parts of the jawbone must be cleaned.

Even though conventional dentists often believe that all of the periodontal ligament, since it is attached to the tooth, comes out with the tooth completely intact, often it does not. If the periodontal ligament is not all removed, the body often does not recognize the tooth is missing. Consequently, proper healing of the anchor points in the surgical site in the jawbone cannot occur. This can cause an open space in the jawbone called a cavitation. Cavitations can quickly become a collecting pool for a focal infection, which, over time, can cause damage and disease in other parts of the body.

Infection in the bone that is not removed doesn't just go away. Dentists often prescribe an antibiotic to remedy this situation, but there is no way to guarantee that the antibiotic will even get to the infected tissue. In addition, an antibiotic wreaks havoc on the immune system, disrupts the natural biome in the gut, and, if not successful in eradicating all the pathogens, can help create more antibiotic-resistant strains of the infection. How much better to remove the infected bone tissue and then treat the area with laser and ozone? Tooth replacement of some type is recommended and is discussed in Chapter 9.

CHAPTER 8

The Dangers of Root-Canal-Treated Teeth

Peter looked at the clock on his nightstand – it was 2 a.m. It was only 10 minutes since he last checked, but it seemed like an hour. What started as a mild toothache had greatly intensified, and the only over-the-counter pain reliever he could tolerate wasn't helping.

Initially, it was a dull pain that would come and go. When it hurt, it was tolerable, so he didn't resort to medication. When the pain would go away, it supported what he wanted to believe: that it was nothing serious. But now, it was no longer tolerable. The dull ache had become a sharp, shooting pain that made him wince.

Reluctantly, he decided to take something for the pain. At that point, he realized his pain had escalated to what was similar to that which his wife had experienced just before she surrendered to having a root canal. He resigned himself to doing what he had hoped to avoid – he would call his dentist, and if his dentist recommended a root canal, he would say, "Go ahead."

Peter's experience is quite typical. Often, when a tooth begins to ache, people will avoid seeking treatment until the pain reaches or exceeds their tolerance level. Then, there is a powerful motivation to make a hurried trip to the dentist. At that point, however, the high level of desperation clouds the decision-making process. They want quick relief, and whatever the dentist suggests is quickly accepted. In the case of a root canal procedure, fast pain relief also comes with probable, long-term health consequences.

This trade-off happens daily in the office of traditional dentists who do not understand the need to maintain a healthy oral terrain. The patient and allopathic dentist see the tooth as an isolated problem that must be addressed without understanding the extensive ecosystem (terrain) that influences the other teeth, the gums, and the jaw bone. These structures are directly connected to several bodily networks, including the vascular and lymphatic systems, that transport healthy and infected fluids throughout the body. In addition, the structures that channel energy throughout the body can be maintained or impeded depending on how this infected tooth is treated.

The "Positive" Side of a Root Canal

A root canal procedure is typically done when the soft pulp tissue inside a tooth becomes infected or inflamed or because a tooth is abscessed. The infection or inflammation can have a variety of causes, such as deep decay, repeated dental procedures on the tooth, a chip, crack, or a fracture in a tooth resulting in exposure of the pulp and nerves. An abscess occurs when pus forms at the root of an infected tooth. Any of these can occur with or without pain or other symptoms.

From a pragmatic viewpoint, a root canal eliminates pain and keeps an attractive, functional chewing surface in the mouth. I cannot deny the positive aspects of this. However, that's far from the whole story.

The Problematic Aspects of a Root Canal
1. It provides a Pain-Free Home for a Dead Tooth

Healthy teeth are alive. They are fed by blood vessels and the lymphatic system and have nerves like other bodily organs and tissues. A root canal procedure removes these connections to "save" the tooth. "Saving the tooth" is a severe misnomer. Either the tooth is dead when the procedure is done, or it will kill the tooth if it is still alive at the beginning of the procedure.

Ultimately, the purpose of the procedure is to keep a dead tooth in the mouth. Think about it: There is no other body part that medical or dental practitioners try to keep attached to the body when it dies. Except for a root-canal-treated tooth, necrotic (dead) tissue is always removed to prevent severe infection and even death.

Blood and lymphatic vessels, nerves, and connective tissues that keep the tooth alive enter the tooth through a small hole in the tip of each root and up through a canal in the soft pulp in the tooth's core. A root canal procedure removes all of the soft pulp, vessels, nerves, and connective tissue by drilling through the top of the tooth, the enamel that covers the exterior part of the tooth, and then through the dentin into the pulp. Then, the drill is used to hollow out the pulp and everything in the canals in each root. In the case of front teeth, generally, there is only one root, while molars usually have two, three, or even four roots.

Then, the hollowed-out chamber is sterilized, presumably to kill ambient bacteria in the tooth. Once deemed to be sterile, the chamber is filled and sealed. This filling material always contains some metal – so the root-canal-treated tooth can be identified on an X-ray. Finally, the tooth is capped with a crown or sometimes a filling.

So, the patient is left with an attractive, functional, pain-free tooth. But this is one of the problems with the root canal procedure. True, a dead tooth feels no pain, but it also can't alert you when there is a severe problem. It is akin to disconnecting a smoke detector because you don't want your sleep interrupted in the middle of the night.

2. It Establishes a Breeding Ground for Pathogens

After a root canal, the dead tooth always becomes an environment conducive to sheltering chronic infection. That's because there is no reliable way to completely sterilize a root-canal-treated tooth (while it is still in a patient's mouth). Until it is extracted and the tooth socket is cleaned, this tooth provides the perfect environment for infections to grow and spread throughout the whole body.

This is why: The body of the tooth, which surrounds the main root canal, consists of tissue called dentin, which is incredibly porous and accounts for about 90 percent of a tooth's structure. Under a microscope, the dentin looks similar to a honeycomb.

This porous tissue comprises a vast, intricate network of microscopically tiny canals called dentin tubules. The dentin tubules run from the main root canal out toward the exterior of the tooth. The dentin tubules serve the purpose of transporting nutrients obtained from blood to all parts of the tooth. The nutrient-rich fluid, or protoplasm, that flows through the dentin tubules is necessary to keep a tooth alive and healthy.

Were all the tubules in a single tooth laid end-to-end, they would extend for several miles. Though microscopically small, the dentin tubules easily accommodate the even smaller bacteria and other microbes, such as streptococcus, staphylococcus, spirochetes, and protozoa. However, because of the surface tension of sterilizing agents, these tubes will not allow the entrance of these agents. Thus, these microbes are given a safe haven.

Root-canal filling materials, disinfecting chemicals, antibiotics, lasers, and ozone therapy can effectively sterilize the hollowed-out pulp chamber. However, these treatments are ineffective at getting into and sterilizing the vast network of dentin tubules where the microbes feed on decaying protoplasm.

Oral antibiotics cannot circulate into the tooth because the tooth's blood supply has been removed. They have no way of getting to the bacteria within a root-canal-treated tooth. Therefore, all root-canal-treated teeth will harbor some bacteria and possibly other microbes, even if done perfectly.

3. It Creates Factories for the Production of Deadly Toxins

A dead, sealed tooth stimulates the adaptation of oxygen-breathing bacteria (aerobic) into non-oxygen-breathing (anaerobic) microbes so these pathogens can survive without oxygen. Undoubtedly, you have heard of botulism. It is caused by the bacterium *Clostridium botulinum*, which is quite common in soil and water. In its aerobic state, this micro-organism is relatively harmless. But when placed in a very low-oxygen environment, these microbes become anaerobic and produce the botulinum toxin, which can be deadly. This is why people must be careful when canning certain vegetables.

In the same way, entombed bacteria in the dentin tubules in a root-canal-treated tooth can become anaerobic and excrete pathogenic poisons called exotoxins or thioethers as their metabolic waste. As this change in their metabolism occurs, the bacteria become smaller, more virulent, and more dangerous. Research has shown that thioethers, which can seep out of the tooth into the bone and gum tissue and eventually into the rest of the body through the bloodstream, can damage the heart, kidneys, lungs, eyes, stomach, brain, and any other parts of the human body.

Health Consequences of Root-Canal-Treated Teeth

Causal links between root-canal-treated teeth and other conditions have been observed and reported. Among these chronic diseases are:

✓ Arthritis

✓ Meningitis

✓ Pneumonia

✓ Appendicitis

✓ Anemia

✓ Heart lesions

✓ Endocarditis, myocarditis (heart inflammation)

✓ Hardening of the arteries

✓ Nervous system breakdowns

✓ Eye infections

✓ Kidney, liver, and gallbladder problems

✓ Cancer

A Couple of Actual Case Reports

"I had my mercury fillings removed and one root canal done. A year later, I developed pain in both hands, and my thumbs were locked in an open position. At this point, I met Dr. Garcia, who encouraged me to have the root canal tooth pulled, indicating a correlation between root canals and rheumatoid arthritis.

"I did not want my tooth pulled, and it took me several days to consider this option. But eventually, I concluded that removing the tooth might help the pain in my hand joints, so I was willing to try. I did have the tooth pulled, and the lab report showed the tooth was infected down to the bone. Since its removal, I have regained the use of my thumbs, and the finger joint pain has diminished.

"Secondly, my husband went through a similar experience. He had had three root canals done close to one another by another dentist before meeting Dr. Garcia, who encouraged my husband to have all three root canals extracted. And once again, all three were infected, and two were abscessed. It is obvious to us both that root canals can be very dangerous, as the dead tissue can feed harmful bacteria to all body parts without you ever knowing.

"Knowing the dangers of root canals, I will never have another one done. Interestingly, there was never any pain or discomfort in the tooth (when I had pain in my hands). Most people would never make the connection between a root canal and disease."

J.W.

Other Obvious Connections

The link between a root-canal-treated tooth and disease in another area of the body was clear in J.W.'s case. Unfortunately, it's a connection that most health-care practitioners and their patients are unaware of.

And yet, the failure to see the relationship is puzzling when you consider that *these same practitioners are quite aware of the correlation between periodontal disease and other health problems because of published research that readily acknowledges the connection.* Many studies have linked periodontitis and conditions such as heart disease, stroke, respiratory diseases, diabetes, osteoporosis, and difficulties during pregnancy.

Periodontal disease is the general label used to describe chronic infection and/or inflammation of the gums and the supporting structures of the teeth. The American Academy of Periodontology seeks to educate the public about research that supports what perceptive dentists inevitably recognize: "Infections in the mouth can play havoc elsewhere in the body." Even though periodontal disease is generally acknowledged as a potential risk factor for other systemic diseases and ailments, the much greater risk posed by root-canal-treated teeth remains inexplicably ignored by conventional dental and medical establishments.

Consequently, every year, millions of Americans undergo at least one root canal procedure with no awareness of the risk to their overall health. Rather than extracting a diseased, dying, or already dead tooth, a root-canal procedure is almost universally the "standard of care" unless patients elect to forego the procedure because of its high cost or have already become aware of the health risks. Despite much evidence to the contrary, the dental establishment endorses root canal procedures as the safe, effective, and preferred treatment for teeth that should be extracted.

The entire endodontic industry in the U.S., which includes nearly 50,000 endodontists plus their support staff, is exclusively devoted to performing root canal procedures. Considerable energy and money are spent annually to defend and promote this dental procedure. Unfortunately, this effort effectively conveys the dangerous misconception that there are no risks involved for their patients.

Most dental practitioners don't realize that a root-canal-treated tooth can directly cause numerous degenerative diseases, including cardiovascular disease, brain and nervous system disorders, kidney disease, rheumatoid arthritis, and even cancer. In addition to potentially being a causative factor for a specific degenerative disease, a root-canal-treated tooth can directly cause various chronic ailments, such as infections, inflammation, pain, blood cell abnormalities, and fatigue.

In America today, many people suffer from diseases or ailments that modern medicine says are of unknown cause (etiology). If you have at least one root-canal-treated tooth, understanding that it can damage your health may help you realize freedom from a disease or ailment you are now experiencing. Increasingly, holistically-minded dentists, physicians, and other practitioners are beginning to realize that many chronic and degenerative diseases and conditions with no conventionally recognized cause can sometimes be cured by extracting root-canal teeth and adequately cleaning the tooth sockets.

Respected Researchers Express Great Concern

The Meticulous Research of Dr. Weston Price

In the early years of the 20th century, holistic dental pioneer and researcher Weston Price and his team of over 60 others made important discoveries regarding root-canal-treated teeth. What I have learned from my clinical experience and research confirms their findings. Dr. Price led a comprehensive long-term project that investigated what happens to a tooth after a root-canal procedure is done to it. During the 25 years of his clinical and laboratory research, he found that a root-canal procedure could produce unexpected and unintended consequences.

This work was documented in 25 articles and two books, published in 1923, and titled *Dental Infections, Oral and Systemic* and *Dental Infections and the Degenerative Diseases*. This comprehensive research teaches us that when a root-canal procedure is done to a tooth, the tooth always becomes an environment conducive to harboring infection. When the condition occurs, the tooth inevitably becomes a source of chronic and insidious stress for the whole body.

Even though Dr. Price was director of the Research Institute of the National Dental Association (now the American Dental Association [ADA]) from 1914 to 1928, and his research was initially supported by the dental establishment of the time, the dental and medical world disregards his research today. The complete dismissal of Dr. Price's findings is inexplicable, as no clinical research shows contrary results.

His research also strongly supported the focal infection theory, which was generally accepted in his day. This theory states that an infection affecting one area of the body can lead to subsequent conditions or symptoms in other areas. This can occur due to the spread of the infectious agent or toxins it produces. Even though most conventional healthcare practitioners reject the focal infection theory, they readily accept a similar phenomenon as they recognize that cancer cells can spread to other organs and tissues via circulating blood.

Before and during the period that Dr. Price and his team were doing their research, microbiology researchers, including those at the famous Mayo Clinic, had determined that over 90 percent of all focal infections came from the teeth and tonsils. However, in the conventional medical and dental realm today, focal infection is accepted only minimally.

If focal infections don't infect other parts of the body, why do conventional dentists prophylactically give antibiotics to patients with certain health conditions before a dental procedure? They recognize that bacteria in the mouth (a focal infection) might get into the bloodstream. At the same time, the most common and potentially dangerous source of focal infection, a root-canal-treated tooth, is never considered a potential health risk.

Details of Price's Clinical Experiences and Research

As a practicing dentist, Dr. Price became suspicious that root-canal-treated teeth were directly causing degenerative diseases in some of his patients. When patients with at least one root canal began to suffer from chronic health problems the medical profession couldn't alleviate, Dr. Price began to consider those root-canal-treated teeth might be a source of infection, causing damage to other tissues in the body.

One day, while treating a woman who had used a wheelchair for six years due to severe arthritis, he investigated whether a chronic infection was brewing in her dead tooth. He advised this patient to have her root canal tooth extracted to determine if it was responsible for her suffering. The extracted tooth looked fine — the filling showed no evidence of infection, and it appeared normal on X-ray pictures. Dr. Price then surgically implanted the tooth beneath the skin of a healthy rabbit. Within 48 hours, the rabbit was crippled with arthritis.

However, once the woman's root-canal-treated tooth was out of her mouth, her arthritic condition improved dramatically. She could walk without a cane and even do fine needlework in a short time. This experiment led Dr. Price to conclude that something about the root-canal-treated tooth caused arthritis in both the woman and the rabbit.

This moved Dr. Price to advise other patients who suffered from diseases that conventional medicine could not help to have their root-canal teeth extracted. The most valuable part of Dr. Price's research was that many patients with root-canal teeth removed recovered from their chronic illnesses, usually within 48 hours. Dr. Price found that various medical conditions, ranging from arthritis to nervous system disorders, could be alleviated by removing root-canal-treated teeth.

Dr. Price repeated his testing procedure with people and lab animals hundreds of times. After extracting a root-canal-treated tooth from a patient, he learned that it didn't matter whether he implanted the entire tooth or only a portion of the tooth under the skin of a lab animal – the same result would occur. The animal would almost always develop the same disease as the patient, and most of the animals died within two weeks because the infections proved so devastating to them. His experiments demonstrated that a root-canal-treated tooth might be a causative factor in systemic disease of both people and animals.

Not only did Dr. Price and his research team discover that a wide variety of degenerative diseases could be transferred to animals using root-canal teeth, but they also found that various bacteria had an affinity for specific tissues and tended to migrate there. If a patient had a heart condition that improved after extraction of a root-canal tooth and that same tooth was implanted into a lab animal, the animal would develop a heart condition. If a patient had kidney trouble, the animal would develop kidney trouble. If the patient had an eye condition, the animal would have difficulty with its eyes.

Toxic Effects Without Bacteria

As their research progressed, Dr. Price and his colleagues developed the practice of obtaining bacteria cultures from root-canal-treated teeth to inject the bacteria into lab animals. This way, they could control the bacteria concentration the animals were exposed to. But even when only a millionth of a gram, or one microgram, of bacteria was injected into an animal, it would still become seriously ill. With such a tiny amount of bacteria involved, Dr. Price questioned whether something other than the bacteria could be hurting the animals.

So, experiments were developed that went like this: An extracted root-canal-treated tooth was crushed, washed, and put in a centrifuge or passed through a special filter to remove bacteria. The remaining solution was tested to ensure all the bacteria had been removed and injected into lab animals. Amazingly, this bacteria-free extract would still cause the animals to get sick and die, often sooner than when an entire tooth was implanted under their skin.

This research showed that it was the toxins produced by the bacteria, rather than the presence of the bacterial infection itself, that caused disease and killed the lab animals. Price's research team theorized that when the bacteria were present, they at least stimulated an immune-system response that helped some of the animals survive longer. The toxins alone did not produce an immune system response.

His research team repeatedly demonstrated that it could reproduce a patient's disease in a lab animal from bacterial toxins and that these toxins had a poisoning effect even in tiny amounts. Also, these toxins remain in the tooth long after the bacteria are gone. So, even if sterilization procedures could completely kill all the bacteria in root-canal teeth, this careful and precise research demonstrated that the potent toxins produced by the bacteria remained in the tooth in amounts that were lethal enough to kill lab animals.

The Primary Microbes Infecting Root Canals

Dr. Price and this research team isolated many bacteria and other microbes from root-canal-treated teeth. They learned that the primary microbes infecting root canals were streptococcus, staphylococcus, and spirochetes. Streptococcus was found more than 90 percent of the time and was often accompanied by other organisms from the staphylococcus and spirochete families. Therefore, a single root-canal tooth can harbor more than one type of infectious organism, and different root-canal teeth can have different bacteria and other microbes.

Bacteriologists have confirmed that these strains of bacteria are commonly found in dental infections (as well as infections in the tongue, throat, and other parts of the oral cavity), but what Dr. Price learned was that each strain of bacteria is capable of producing diseases in other parts of the body, depending on the nature of the particular organism. And because there usually is more than one type of bacteria residing in a root-canal tooth, and there may be two or more root-canal teeth, a person can become simultaneously afflicted with the symptoms of more than one disease or ailment.

Although Dr. Price and his team learned that the bacteria and toxins from root-canal teeth could cause harm to any area of the body, the heart, circulatory system, and blood cells were most commonly affected. Heart and circulatory conditions, together with blood cell abnormalities, that could be caused by the toxins coming from root-canal-treated teeth were endocarditis, myocarditis, pericarditis, heart blockage, aortitis, angina pectoris, phlebitis, arteriosclerosis, hypertension, hypotension, anemia, leucopenia, leukocytosis, lymphopenia, lymphocytosis, and bacteremia.

The next most common were joint diseases, such as arthritis, and diseases of the brain and nervous system. The bacterial toxins from root-canal teeth also damage the kidneys, eyes, lungs, liver, gallbladder, neck, back, shoulder, ears, shins, appendix, ovaries, testes, and bladder.

Even though this research was done between 1900 and 1925, it is as valuable now as it was. Dr. Price and his research team repeated experiments hundreds of times to ensure accurate and reproducible results. Any dentist who practices with holistic awareness will learn from their own experience that Dr. Price made vital discoveries about the root-canal procedure. A no-nonsense way of describing what I believe is the main lesson of Dr. Price's root-canal research is this: Dead teeth do not belong in live bodies.

The Insights of Dr. Josef Issels

Throughout the 1930s and 1940s, a doctor and surgeon named Josef Issels became increasingly dissatisfied with conventional medicine's approach to treating cancer. He knew there had to be a better way to help people than treating their tumor sites with surgery, radiation, or poisons, euphemistically called chemotherapy. He knew these medical treatments did nothing to determine why people got cancer in the first place.

After years of research, the holistic-minded Dr. Issels concluded that "cancer is a general disease of the whole body" rather than a local disease confined to where a tumor occurs. Dr. Issels saw cancer as a chronic, systemic illness and the tumor as a late-stage symptom "able to exist and grow only in a 'bed' already prepared for it." The "bed" he referred to was an internal environment resulting from metabolic disturbances and damage to the body's organs and systems, ultimately weakening the body's natural defenses against malignancy. He called this the "tumor milieu."

Awareness of this insight is necessary to understand that the treatment that offers the best chance for success in overcoming cancer treats "not merely the tumor but also the whole body, which has produced the tumor."

During his research, Dr. Issels learned that focal infections, such as root-canal-treated teeth, could be a source of stress for a person's immune system. He believed that the stress and toxicity from a focal infection could weaken the body's ability to maintain homeostasis (balance) and be a significant causative factor in the development of many diseases, including cancer.

In 1947, Dr. Issels began implementing a comprehensive "whole body" approach to helping people overcome cancer. Over the next 40 years, he treated over 16,000 people, most of whom had advanced cancers. Unlike doctors who used only conventional treatments, Dr. Issels achieved an impressively high remission rate, especially with late-stage cancer patients. These were patients whom traditional doctors regarded as "terminal and hopeless."

Although Dr. Issels emphasized nutrition and treated the whole person, including a patient's emotional issues, a fundamental part of his treatment was that he required all his patients to have any root-canal teeth extracted. He also insisted that any other dead or infected teeth be extracted.

Dr. Issels learned that about 90 percent of his cancer patients had between two and ten dead teeth in their mouths when they first arrived at his clinic for treatment. In his book *Cancer: A Second Opinion*, published in 1975, Dr. Issels wrote of his research on root-canal-treated teeth and said that dead teeth left in the mouth could become toxin factories because the bacteria in these teeth do produce thioethers. Dr. Issels believed that thioethers produced by anaerobic bacteria in root-canal-treated teeth had all the properties of a substance capable of causing cancer and other diseases in people.

The Contribution of Dr. Thomas Rau

Much more recently, the holistic-minded Dr. Thomas Rau, who heads the Paracelsus Clinic in Switzerland, had this to say about root-canal teeth and women he has treated with breast cancer:

"I made a study of breast cancer patients and found that 98 percent had a disturbance on the stomach (acupuncture) meridian. (The breast belongs to the same acupuncture meridian.) These patients have a typical psychological background pattern and disturbances of their stomach meridian. In 150 cases of women with breast cancer, we only had three patients who did not have a root canal in a tooth that belonged to the stomach acupuncture meridian. You see, each tooth belongs to a meridian, and 98 percent (of the women with breast cancer) had a root canal (tooth) on the same meridian that belongs to the breast. It's exciting.

"Of course, when I brought this up in a medical congress, they simply said, 'Well, in this day and age, all women have root canals.' So, we did a study of women in the same age range without breast cancer without chronic diseases, and only 30 percent of that group had root canals. It's a significant difference.

"I'm not saying that root canals cause breast cancer, but if you have breast cancer and you don't remove your root canals and the other toxic elements that bother the breast tissue, then you have a lower chance to heal."

Dr. George Meinig Discovers the Research of Dr. Weston Price

Dr. George Meinig founded the American Association of Endodontists (root canal specialists) in Chicago in 1943. During his 47 years of practice, Dr. Meinig did countless root canals and taught the procedure at dental association workshops nationwide. Unfortunately, it wasn't until after Dr. Meinig retired that he discovered the extensive research of Dr. Weston Price on the consequences of root canals.

Dr. Meinig explained: "While reading all 1,174 pages of the two volumes of Dr. Price's ... research, I immediately realized ... that Dr. Price's research was thorough and sound. It was easy to see why he was revered as a dental-research specialist. The gist of the research and the thousands of animal studies is this: That root-canal-filled teeth always remain infected no matter how good they might look or how good they might feel."

Dr. Meinig was shocked that the dental establishment entirely disregarded Dr. Price's research. During all the years that Dr. Meinig had been doing and teaching the root canal procedure, he was unaware that it could be damaging to a patient's overall health. He had never even considered the possibility. No other dentist or endodontist that he knew considered the possibility, either. After all, Dr. Price's research was never mentioned in any dental school curriculum, and conventional medicine ignored it.

It was evident to Dr. Meinig that the studies of Dr. Price and his team of researchers had been suppressed by what he called "the autocratic action of a small (but very influential) group of dentists and physicians who refused to accept the focal infection theory." Remember that the focal infection theory states that an infection in one area of the body can lead to diseases or symptoms in other areas of the body due either to the spread of the infectious agent itself or the toxins produced by it.

To once again quote Dr. Meinig: "Despite the experiments conducted on 5,000 animals, and despite the thoroughness and excellence of his root-canal research, all of Price's 25 years of scientific efforts were so well covered up that there is hardly a (conventional) dentist alive today who has ever heard about his discoveries.

"You are all aware that many great medical discoveries sometimes take years and years of research to locate the organism causing the disease. In almost all cases, it is one organism causing one disease. Dr. Price found that at least 20 organisms were responsible for infections in the teeth. These 20 organisms caused not one disease but several oral and dental illnesses. But more importantly, these germs are responsible for many medical diseases manifesting in other body parts."

To begin educating dentists, endodontists, other healthcare practitioners, and the public about Dr. Price's work, Dr. Meinig wrote a book called *Root Canal Cover-Up*, published in 1994. Until he died in 2008, at 93, Dr. Meinig dedicated himself to giving media interviews and public lectures to warn of the dangers of root canals.

Essential Questions About Root Canals

Why Do I Have Such a High Regard for Dr. Price's Work

While most dentists and physicians do not highly regard Dr. Price, I do. Throughout my years as a holistic dentist, I have been interested in how a person's overall health can be affected by the procedures and materials used in dentistry. That intense interest led me to read Dr. Price's books over 24 years ago.

Although a growing number of researchers and holistic-minded practitioners who address the root canal/disease connection have confirmed the validity of Price's research, what matters most to me is that my clinical experience has consistently supported what he discovered many years ago.

Our personal experience can be one of our most valuable teachers (if we are truly paying attention), and my own clinical experience has supported Dr. Price's discoveries and conclusions in the following ways:

First, whenever I have removed the crown or filling from a root-canal-treated tooth, there is always a release of a sick, putrefying odor – it stinks! Then, upon examining the tooth, it is always dry and brittle. The putrefying odor, dryness, and brittleness are expected from anything dead and decomposed by aggressive strains of microbes.

Next, any time I have extracted a root-canal-treated tooth and then sent it to a lab for analysis, the report has consistently confirmed that the tooth was infected. Most importantly, I have seen many patients who have experienced varying degrees of relief from diseases or ailments after having a root-canal tooth or teeth extracted and the tooth socket(s) adequately cleaned.

Before I complete this treatise against the root-canal procedure, I want to acknowledge that a root-canal-treated tooth does not **always**, or even usually, cause a chronic ailment or degenerative disease. However, I aim to help readers understand that a root-canal-treated tooth **can** directly cause chronic illnesses and degenerative diseases. Most healthcare practitioners do not even consider this possibility because they are unaware of it or have disregarded it.

When authority figures in dentistry or medicine say there is no connection between a root-canal-treated tooth and the onset of an ailment or disease, they are admitting that they have not looked for such a connection. And so, it does not exist for them because they will not find it if they do not look!

I do not doubt that many people suffer from various ailments and diseases directly caused by the infection and toxicity of root-canal-treated teeth.

Do All Root-Canal-Treated Teeth Cause Disease?

Some people can be healthy and strong enough to overcome the infection and toxicity from root-canal-treated teeth. A "big picture" understanding comes down to this: Whether or when someone experiences adverse results after undergoing a root-canal procedure is primarily determined, like all aspects of our health, by the dynamic interaction between our genes and our environment (both internal and external).

So, if you have "good genes" and, in particular, a robust immune system (to overcome infection), as well as a strong liver (to detoxify toxins), along with enough good eating habits to support your immune system and liver, and you can avoid intolerable levels of stress, you may be able to prevent any adverse effects of a root canal.

Over a lifetime, however, we will all encounter stressful events that can challenge or overwhelm our body's ability to maintain homeostasis (balance). Our bodies then become susceptible to the effects of a germ or toxin we previously could handle.

It's a biological fact that each person has a unique capacity to tolerate acute or chronic stress. With chronic stress, there is a wear-and-tear effect. The longer a body is stressed with an infection and toxicity from a root-canal-treated tooth, the more likely the body's ability to maintain homeostasis will be compromised. When someone experiences a root-canal-caused ailment or disease many years after the procedure, the thought that a root-canal tooth could be the direct cause won't be considered by a conventional practitioner, so the facts won't be discovered unless the patient finds a holistic practitioner or learns about the possible consequences of a root canal on their initiative.

There is also no doubt that many people with robust enough immune systems and livers capable of efficient detoxification activity can live symptom-free with a root-canal-treated tooth or teeth for many years. However, if someone's immune system and liver are significantly weakened by mercury leeching from

amalgam fillings, environmental pollution, poor nutrition, lack of sleep, chronic stress, toxic medical treatments, alcoholism or other types of substance abuse,
physical or emotional trauma, that person's body may
no longer be able to handle the insidious infection
and toxicity that are almost inevitable consequences of
having a root canal.

Hasn't There Been Progress in the Root Canal Procedure Since Dr. Price's Time?

The short answer is "Yes." Over the past 90-plus
years since Dr. Price completed his research on root-canal-treated teeth, new techniques, and materials have
been used for the procedure, and powerful antibiotics
that were not available in Dr. Price's time are part of
modern medicine and dentistry's arsenal for killing
the infection. But despite all this seemingly significant
progress, an ever-growing body of evidence derived from
recent research and clinical experience strongly supports
the same conclusions Dr. Price arrived at. More specifically, current research done with an electron microscope
has verified that a root-canal-treated tooth does harbor
anaerobic bacteria, which is the basis for how a root-
canal tooth can be a direct causative factor in disease.

Also, to re-emphasize what I said earlier, research
supported by the American Academy of Periodontology
has led to the understanding that "infections in the
mouth can play havoc elsewhere in the body."
Unfortunately, periodontists are focused only on the
gums and the supporting structures of the teeth. But what

about the teeth themselves? And, in particular, teeth subjected to the highly invasive root-canal procedure? Doesn't it seem reasonable to directly consider the teeth as sources of infections in the mouth that can negatively impact other parts of the body?

Are There Any Good Alternatives to the Root Canal Procedure?

Unfortunately, there are no ideal alternatives at this time. Every individual needs to evaluate their situation and consider the upside and downside of each available option.

If you decide that undergoing a root-canal procedure is worth risking possible damage to your overall health, consider the root-canal-treated tooth as no more than a temporary solution for your present circumstances. Having it in your plans to remove the tooth at an appropriate time should be seriously considered, especially if you develop a specific health problem or experience a noticeable decrease in energy and an increase in your susceptibility to feeling ill after the root canal procedure. Remember always to pay attention to your dental history when considering the cause of a seemingly unrelated health problem.

What Should You Do If You Have One or More Root-Canal-Treated Teeth?

Even though I am deeply opposed to the root-canal procedure, I do not automatically conclude that a root-canal-treated tooth should always and immediately be extracted, nor did Dr. Weston Price. So, with this in mind, if you do have at least one root canal tooth but are currently free from any chronic health problem, your answers to the following questions should be carefully considered before deciding that you want to have any root canal tooth or teeth extracted:

- ✓ Are you satisfied with your current state of health?

- ✓ What goals do you have for your health?

- ✓ How committed are you to removing obstacles to an optimum state of health?

- ✓ What is your dental history?

- ✓ What is your medical history?

- ✓ What is your immediate family's dental and medical history?

Suppose you have at least one root-canal-treated tooth and one chronic health problem or degenerative disease. In that case, all of the above questions plus several additional questions require detailed answers before deciding that you want to have any root-canal tooth or teeth extracted:

- ✓ Did you become aware of the ailment or disease after having a root canal procedure?

- ✓ Have the recommended treatments failed?

- ✓ Have conventional or alternative healthcare practitioners failed to find the cause?

Now, for anyone with at least one root-canal-treated tooth and who also suffers from any ailment or disease that they began to notice after having the root-canal procedure, the most valuable part of Dr. Price's research was the discovery that the extraction of the root-canal tooth could often completely alleviate the ailment or disease.

Extracting a tooth is serious; not everyone experiences dramatic or significant improvements after extracting a root-canal tooth. Of course, there can be several other causative factors in a chronic ailment or disease, and the infection and toxicity of a root canal tooth is only one possible cause. But because it is one probable cause, it should be considered.

On the surface, having a root canal procedure instead of extracting a tooth is appealing. A tooth is an essential part of your body that you don't want to lose. But seeing your health holistically is vital so you can avoid losing much more than a tooth! It's silly for us to think of ourselves as a collection of body parts that function independently of each other—holistically, seeing your health leads to understanding that every aspect of your body can influence the whole.

Summing Up: The Risk of Root Canals

Millions of people suffer from chronic illnesses for which the medical profession cannot find a cause or cure. But the "treatments" prescribed to manage these illnesses continue bankrupting our society. Although

I acknowledge exceptional circumstances in which a root canal has short-term value, I believe that phasing out the procedure as a standard-of-care practice would significantly reduce the number of chronic illnesses that burden the American people.

Conventional dentists and physicians won't consider the possibility of a connection between a root-canal-treated tooth and a disease or ailment, especially when the root canal was done many years before symptoms of the disease or condition were noticed. So, if you have a health problem or disease that began after you had one or more root-canal procedures, you will most likely have to urge your dentist or physician to consider such a connection. If they dismiss the possibility, you should seek out other practitioners who are informed about this issue. One of my patients, LV, did just that and avoided two unnecessary medical procedures.

After undergoing a root canal procedure in her lower right molar, LV continued to experience discomfort. The dentist who did the root canal told her that was impossible because all the nerves had been removed from the tooth. He said to her that the problem must be in an adjacent tooth. He suggested another root canal for the adjacent tooth, but LV was reluctant to agree to this second procedure after her painful experience with the first.

LV then developed a seemingly unrelated lump on her right eyelid. At first, it wasn't enjoyable, and she would camouflage it with makeup and sunglasses, but after a while, it increased in size to the point where it became disfiguring. She understandably became very self-conscious about it.

LV consulted several medical professionals. She wanted to know what the lump was, what could have caused it, and what non-surgical steps could be taken to reduce or remove it. LV said, "No doctor had any specific answers other than 'it's just a fatty lump; these sometimes pop up for no reason. Surgery is the only solution, and there's no guarantee that it won't just come back.' I was soooo not satisfied."

During LV's first consultation with me, I saw that her dental history included the recently done root canal procedure. When LV told me the lump had shown up after the root canal, I suspected it could be her body's response to a pocket of bacteria traveling from the root canal site.

When LV said she was still feeling discomfort, I explained that it was an indication that the infection in the root canal tooth had spread to the specific part of the bone where the tooth was anchored. I suggested to LV that she have the root canal tooth pulled as soon as possible. She did, and within a month, the size of the lump had decreased by about half. Within two months, the lump disappeared entirely, and the pain stopped.

LV's story supports what Dr. Weston Price discovered many years ago: Leaving a dead tooth in a patient's mouth can put them at increased risk of various health problems. So, if a dentist recommends a root canal procedure to "save" your tooth from being pulled, remember to ask yourself, "How will I be affected if I have a dead, chronically infected tooth in my mouth?"

CHAPTER 9

Why and How Should Extracted Teeth be Replaced?

Replacement Rationale

The most common and yet least important reason for replacing missing teeth is that having gaping holes in your mouth is unattractive. That's not to say we shouldn't want a beautiful set of ivories beaming through our smiles. Of course, this is a valid consideration, but our long-term health and well-being are much more critical.

Missing Teeth Disrupt a Healthy Terrain

Our bodies were designed to live in balance. This principle affects our ability to walk, run, jump, and dance. It is also critical in our ability to see and hear. We often talk about balance regarding our emotions and our mind. In like manner, It doesn't take much study to notice the order and harmony of a healthy set of teeth. From side to side, there are perfect matches; from top to bottom, every tooth has an opposing mate.

This requirement of body balance, specifically in the mouth, extends beyond appearance and chewing function – although these are undoubtedly important. When you purchase a new set of tires for your car, the installer is supposed to "balance" the wheels before putting them back on your vehicle. Why? Because the vibration caused by spinning tires that are not balanced can cause damage to other parts of the car.

In a much more dramatic way, a mouth with one or more missing teeth has consequences far beyond what we see or think. An unbalanced mouth affects the flow of blood, lymphatic fluids, nerve impulses, and energy. The jaw bone under a missing tooth loses bone density. Unopposed molars tend to move away from the jawbone, exposing part of the tooth without enamel and normally covered by gum tissue to potential decay. Chewing to avoid missing teeth impacts your jaw muscles and other supporting structures.

These consequences, and unnamed others, negatively affect a body's ability to defend itself from opportunistic forces or organisms – in other words, they disrupt a healthy terrain.

Choosing Materials that Promote a Healthy Terrain

All Metals Should Be Avoided

All metals cause some degree of galvanic stress for four reasons:

1. Because of their nature, metals can produce an electrical current in the mouth. This phenomenon only requires two or more dissimilar metals and saliva, which acts like an electrolyte solution.

2. That current causes corrosion and abrasion.

3. Metals often provoke allergic reactions and autoimmune dysfunction.

4. They adversely affect the flow of energy through channels of our body known as meridians.

Are There Good Tooth-Replacement Alternatives?

Several health-promoting alternatives for replacing teeth are attractive and functional. These include:

✓ **Metal-free partials** (a removable partial denture): a replacement tooth attached to a base that is "clipped" to the adjoining natural teeth like a puzzle piece; it can be removed for cleaning and easily reinserted.

✓ **Metal-Free Bridges**: a replacement tooth permanently joined to adjacent teeth; the neighboring teeth on each side are crowned, and the false tooth is fused between these crowns (thereby "bridging" the teeth together).

✓ **Metal-Free Implants**: an artificial root that is
permanently implanted into the jawbone. It
serves as a support structure for a metal-free
crown.

Each of these replacement alternatives will be
discussed in separate sections below.

SPECIAL NOTE: If your chosen tooth replacement
involves the extraction of a root-canal-treated tooth, I
strongly recommend that you seek a holistic or a biological dentist. Just pulling the tooth is not enough. The
dentist must adequately clean out the extraction site to
prevent a cavitation, a hole in the jawbone caused by
chronic infection.

Partials

One approach to consider would be extracting a
root-canal-treated tooth and replacing it with either a
biocompatible partial removable denture (a "partial").
A 'partial' is an artificial tooth or teeth attached to a
synthetic material base that is then "clipped" to the
adjoining natural teeth like a puzzle piece. A partial
can be used to replace several missing teeth. While
partials must be removed daily for proper cleaning, they
are easily reinserted. As you might expect, traditional
partials are made on shiny metal frameworks with shiny
metal clasps. So, if you choose to have a partial, emphasize that you want the partials' framework and clasps to
be free of any shiny metal.

There are two advantages to this approach to tooth replacement. First, partials are considerably less expensive than a bridge or an implant. And secondly, unlike a bridge that requires drilling to reshape the tooth or teeth to which the bridge will be anchored, no other teeth in the mouth will be subjected to that kind of trauma. This solution will also give unopposed teeth the necessary biting/chewing surface (if kept in during eating) and the critical spacer forces to keep other teeth from moving.

There are a couple of downsides to a partial:

1. You have the inconvenience factor of removal and replacement. They should be removed at night.

2. They must be cleaned after every meal to avoid a buildup of food and pathogens that can cause decay in the teeth that hold the partial in place.

Bridges

A bridge is a replacement tooth permanently cemented to adjacent teeth. The neighboring teeth on each side are drilled down and fitted with dental crowns, and the false tooth is fused between them (thereby "bridging" the teeth together). The apparent disadvantage of a bridge is that it requires crowning the adjacent teeth even if they are perfectly healthy.

Preparing a tooth for a crown always involves removing all the tooth's enamel and a good portion of dentin, leaving it vulnerable and can compromise its long-term health. If you choose to have a bridge, emphasize that you want the crowns and bridge framework made only of porcelain or ceramic material. If you don't, you will most likely get a porcelain-fused-to-shiny-metal bridge, which only looks like an all-porcelain replacement.

One of my patients experienced dramatic breathing improvements after removing her porcelain-fused-to-metal bridge. When she came to see me, she had decay under the bridge, so I cleaned out the decay and replaced the bridge with an all-zirconia one. Since metals in the mouth can cause allergies, which lead to asthma and difficulty breathing, the change in the "terrain" of her mouth relieved the problem, and the metallic taste disappeared.

Implants

Let's start with the basics. If you've heard of dental implants but aren't quite sure what they are, a dental implant is the part (post) of an artificial tooth that anchors into the jawbone. It is surgically implanted to serve as the supporting structure for a crown. After a few months, when the implant has been integrated into the bone, a crown is cemented on the implant. The crown then serves as the functional replacement for a tooth lost due to injury or disease or extracted for health reasons.

The use of implants has become popular with dentists and their patients since this treatment became widely available in the 1980s, and it has become increasingly common for dental patients to have at least one. But an implant-based artificial tooth also has a downside. Although it doesn't require the crowning of adjacent teeth or the maintenance necessary for a partial-removable denture, it involves implanting a foreign material into the jawbone, and complications can arise from this surgical procedure, especially in someone not in good health. Also, titanium alloy metal implants, the most common type used, can potentially harm our overall health for one or more of the same reasons that elemental, shiny metal restorations can. Here is a quick review of those reasons:

The Problems with Titanium

As a holistic dentist, I have concerns about how implanting any dental material into my patients' jawbones can affect their long-term health. My biggest concern, however, is for patients with implants made of a titanium-based alloy.

As I explained in Chapter 2, I have found that our long-term health should have dental materials made of ceramic or porcelain rather than from shiny metals. However, the most commonly used dental implants continue to be titanium alloys, which are the shiny metal titanium combined with a small but significant amount of other shiny metals, such as aluminum and vanadium.

Along with its use in dental implants, titanium is used in dentistry for orthodontic brackets (braces). Medically, titanium is used for pacemakers, stents, orthopedic implants, and artificial joints. Since titanium is used for all these dental and medical devices, it's easy to assume it must be safe.

From the perspective of conventional dentistry and medicine, titanium is "safe enough." It is strong and durable, and it is relatively easy to use. It integrates with the bone as an implant material and "gets the job done." And because titanium implants usually do not cause acute health problems, they make an excellent first impression on patients and practitioners.

However, from a holistic perspective, titanium alloys may cause or contribute to chronic health problems. Although the advocates promote it as a biologically inert metal, titanium implants release metal ions into the body continuously, which can catalyze galvanic activity, as discussed earlier. In addition, it is well known in dentistry that titanium implants can cause a problem known as peri-implantitis – involving inflammation in the gum tissue and the bone around an implant – which may result in bone loss and eventual implant loss.

According to some leading periodontists, peri-implantitis is nearly pandemic as implants have become more popular with patients and dentists. The dental community admits that peri-implantitis is becoming commonplace and is much more challenging to treat than periodontitis. Considering the downsides of all tooth replacement options, I believe it is important to work diligently to keep living teeth in a patient's mouth as long as possible. The best strategy limits tooth disturbance (drilling, extractions, and movement) as much as possible. While interruption of the natural terrain is avoided, encouraging lifestyle habits that will keep the body and mouth in balance are encouraged. This is the best approach for maintaining health and reducing the need for redoing dental work in the future.

Another complication of the use of titanium is its potential to induce the abnormal proliferation of cells (neoplasia), which can lead to the development of malignant tumors. While rare, it is an acknowledged complication of orthopedic surgery involving titanium hardware implantation.

Returning to oral galvanism, or galvanic stress, I think it's important to briefly review and re-emphasize this phenomenon and how it can affect our health. Oral galvanism is the term used to describe electricity created in the mouth when two or more dissimilar metals are bathed in saliva, which acts as an electrolyte solution. A person's mouth can become much like a car battery as the dissimilar metals react with the electricity-conducting potential of saliva.

The titanium alloy implant (made of more than one metal) can cause galvanic stress. But then, when you add the metals typically used to make the crown, you have even more galvanic stress. If you also have other metal dental work in your mouth, the galvanic stress will increase even more.

The more metal ions react with cells and tissues, the more likely the immune system will develop an allergic response to that metal. A continuously produced unnatural electrical current in the mouth (though very small) will be a source of stress for all the soft tissues in the mouth, like the gums, inner cheeks, and tongue. This constant galvanic stress can lead to such symptoms as:

✓ Inflamed and sore areas in the mouth

✓ A metallic or salty taste or even a burning

sensation in the mouth

✓ Nerve shocks

✓ Ulcerations

✓ Discoloration of the teeth and gums

Unfortunately, dental and medical establishments have very little interest in considering the implications of oral galvanism. But with a holistic understanding of health, looking for a more biocompatible alternative to titanium is natural. This brings us to zirconia.

Why Zirconia Is Better

Zirconia is a fully oxidized form of the element zirconium. It is also known as zirconium oxide ($ZrO2$). Although zirconium is classified as a metal on the Periodic Table of Elements – right below titanium – when it is chemically bonded to oxygen, its properties dramatically change. Functionally, it is now considered a ceramic. Except for retaining its strength and durability, it no longer has the properties of shiny metal. Among other changes, this transformed zirconium salt can no longer generate or conduct an electrical current.

When zirconium is bound to oxygen, it becomes part of an inert crystalline lattice structure. That means it does not allow free metal ions to dissociate and eventually cause trouble for our bodies. Zirconia is, without question, the most immuno-compatible dental implant material available. In addition, it exhibits exceptional strength, durability, resistance to fracture, and its bright, tooth-like color and biocompatibility. In other words, it is the healthier choice for dental-implant material.

For over 20 years, zirconia has been used in the production of hip joint prostheses (artificial joints), and this success has led to a demand for zirconia-based dental implants.

Is an Implant Right for You?

From the perspective of holistic dentistry, several factors should be considered in deciding whether someone is a good candidate for a dental implant. These factors are summarized in the chart below.

Factors That Make Success More Likely:

- ✓ Enough good-quality bone at the implant site
- ✓ Generally good health
- ✓ A "clean" mouth (No source of chronic infection and toxicity)
- ✓ Good nutritional habits
- ✓ Good oral hygiene habits
- ✓ Good sleep habits
- ✓ No self-destructive behavior
- ✓ A skilled dentist
- ✓ Compliance with post-surgical instructions

Factors That Increase the Risk of Failure:

- ✓ Insufficient quantity of good-quality bone at the implant site
- ✓ Generally poor health

✓ A "dirty" mouth (one or more sources of chronic infection and toxicity)

✓ Poor nutritional habits

✓ Poor oral hygiene habits

✓ Smoking

✓ Bruxism (tooth clenching or grinding)

✓ Metabolic and hormonal disorders (especially diabetes)

✓ Chronic sleep deprivation

✓ Auto-immune diseases

✓ Abuse of alcohol and drugs

Other Factors to Consider:

Regarding good nutrition, which is essential for a successful implant, my experience has taught me that people with generally poor eating habits and who strictly follow a vegan, vegetarian diet are especially susceptible to experiencing a loss of mineral density in their jawbone. And if the jawbone doesn't have sufficient density, it becomes brittle and will not hold the implant well.

The artificial root of all dental implants looks like a post or a screw. Because a zirconia implant has a bright, tooth-like color, it has a more pleasing look than the metallic color of a titanium implant.

Even though a dental implant can fuse with the jawbone, it feels different from a natural tooth during chewing. That's because there is no periodontal ligament – the connective tissue – between the implant and the bone. This vital structure acts like a "shock absorber" for the compressive forces during chewing.

After an implant is surgically placed into the jawbone, a healing period is required to allow the implant to fuse to the bone in a process called "osse-ointegration." The time necessary for this fusion can vary significantly from patient to patient, so this issue must be carefully considered. My experience with zirconia implants has taught me that four months should be allowed.

If the implant is "stressed" before it has had time to integrate into the bone, it can move and fail. Then, the subsequent time necessary for the jawbone to heal (with or without a bone graft) in preparation for a new implant may take a year or even longer. So, along with being necessary, allowing enough time for osseointegration to occur offers a chance to develop patience!

Despite the popularity of dental implants with many patients, if you are already challenged with more than minor health issues, it's wise to work on improving your overall health before asking your body to accept a dental implant.

Final Thoughts

In our march toward having more and more technology in our lives, we have created an increasingly artificial environment. We have been, and continue to be, exposed to a wide variety of toxic metals and chemical pollutants daily. These environmental contaminants are found in our air, water, food, and ultimately in us. Toxic metals and chemical pollutants are recognized as causative factors in our population's increasing frequency of allergies, autoimmune diseases, and cancer.

However, because the treatment of dysfunction and chronic disease is mainly in the hands of the medical profession, the potential effects that some dental procedures and materials have on these problems have yet to be noticed, or even ignored, by both conventional dentists and conventional physicians.

People blessed with a robust immune system may be able to neutralize the stress from shiny metal dental work for most or even all of their lives. Still, for people who are not so blessed, I suspect it is only a matter of time before their health is compromised to some degree by the toxic and galvanic stress of dental work made from shiny metals.

Your liver and immune system are working overtime to neutralize the toxins in the air you breathe, the water you drink, the food you eat, and the products you put in your body. Shiny metal ions and molecules from dental materials such as fillings, crowns, and bridges may also burden your immune system. So if you need to replace a missing tooth, a severely injured tooth, or a tooth that you plan to have extracted after previously trying a root-canal procedure, your overall health will benefit from choosing the more innovative and safer zirconia implant instead of the conventional one made from shiny metals.

Conventional dentists and their patients seem to believe it's "normal" to keep adding titanium implants without considering how the whole body will be affected. But it's certainly worth your time to consider these factors. We have only one body to live with in this life. If you don't take care of it, who will?

CHAPTER 10

Getting Your Nutrition Right

NOTE: *This chapter was written with much nutrition advice from Jim Marlowe, the most knowledgeable and brilliant nutritionist I know.* His contribution was so substantial, that when I refer to myself in this chapter it could easily be written as "we" or even "Jim."

Regarding what I know is a fundamentally important under-standing of human metabolism and nutrition, I would also like to express our appreciation for the contributions made by Dr. George Watson, Dr. William Donald Kelley, Dr. Rudolf Wiley and, especially, William Wolcott. I also appreciate the work of Dr. Nicholas Gonzalez, Dr. Harold Kristal and Dodie Anderson.

Introduction

In Chapter 2, I used a garden analogy to explain maintaining a healthy terrain. To carry that further, imagine you want to grow some nutritious fruits or vegetables in your garden. You could 1) throw a ton of chemical fertilizer on the dirt or 2) feed the soil with some organic compost. It's a rhetorical question, but which would be best and why?

At the same time, you would want to avoid contaminating the soil with pesticides and herbicides because, eventually, the roots of your plants will take up those toxins. Getting your nutrition right is much the same. Suppose you are interested in a holistic approach to your health. In that case, you realize that nutrition – what you take into your body – plays a significant role in maintaining a healthy terrain and providing your body with quality building materials.

You know proper nutrition is crucial for your heart, liver, lungs, and kidneys. But what about your dental health? It's just as essential for your teeth and other structures in your mouth.

The Foundational Research of Dr. Price

In addition to his long-term research on root canals, Dr. Weston Price spent many years studying how nutritional practices affect dental and overall health. What follows are some of his fundamental teachings.

During the early part of the 20th century, significant changes occurred in the eating habits of an increasing number of Americans. New and more efficient food processing methods were being developed, and as a result, more and more companies were producing and marketing processed foods. The convenience, shelf life, taste, price, and clever advertisements for these foods attracted more and more Americans to buy them.

Then as now, refined sugar, in some form, is a common ingredient in many processed foods. The consumption of sugar and sugary foods increased substantially during this period. Regarding this trend, some highly relevant historical information can be found in the first United States Department of Agriculture (USDA) food guide, Food for Young Children, published in 1916. In it, sugars and sugary foods were identified as one of the five food groups upon which dietary recommendations were made.[1]

As it became increasingly common for American adults and children to consume sugar and sugary, processed foods, Dr. Price considered the possibility that the change in eating habits from "traditional" foods to "modernized" foods was, to some degree, responsible for the increasing prevalence of tooth decay, crowded, crooked teeth, and malformed dental arches and facial bones that he was seeing in his patients and the American population in general.

To confirm his suspicions, Dr. Price began researching the causes of tooth decay during the late 1920s. Because he was a diligent researcher, his investigation included the influence of different eating habits on dental health. Since he was already familiar with the dental health of people routinely eating varying amounts of refined and processed foods, he wanted to compare their dental health with those eating local, traditional foods. He knew there might be a few such communities of American and Canadian Indians. Still, he wanted to study other communities, so he traveled to different parts of the world to study people who did not eat "modernized foods of commerce" (white sugar, white flour, and other refined and processed foods).

1. Hunt, C.L. Food for Young Children. U.S. Department of Agriculture, Farmers' Bulletin No. 717, 21 pp., 1916.

Throughout the 1930s, Dr. Price studied people in 14 relatively isolated cultures. All of these cultures comprised two distinct communities: those that followed the traditional dietary practices and those that abandoned the practices in favor of refined and processed foods (when such foods became available). In addition to studying communities of Indians living in Florida, Canada, and Alaska, he lived with communities in Switzerland, Africa, Australia, New Zealand, South America, and on Archipelagos in the South Pacific and off the coast of Scotland.

In the 14 cultures he studied, primary attention was paid to the people who still practiced traditional ways of hunting, catching, planting, gathering, and preparing the foods that nature provided. Because he was especially interested in the volume of vitamins and minerals they consumed, he collected representative samples of foods from each culture's traditional and modernized communities. He then analyzed these foods for their vitamin and mineral content.

Although there were substantial differences in the foods eaten by the 14 communities that followed their traditions (they were, of course, dependent on what was available to them), they shared the following general characteristics:

1. They all had "nourishing traditions" – nutritional practices based on experience and handed down from generation to generation. These traditions were all about eating nutrient-dense, wholesome foods that came directly from nature within the area in which they lived.

2. They did not eat any refined and processed, nutrient-depleted and adulterated food products, such as artificially solidified oils known as margarine and shortening, white sugar, white flour, and foods that came in cans, jars, or boxes.

3. They ate both animal-derived and plant-derived foods but in highly variable amounts. There were no nourishing traditions that included only animal-derived foods, and there were no nourishing traditions that included only plant-derived foods. (There were no vegans or vegetarians!)

4. The foods that comprised each culture's nourishing traditions were substantially more nutrient dense than the "modernized foods of commerce." More specifically, when Dr. Price analyzed the samples of foods that he collected from both the traditional and modernized communities in each culture, he identified the following differences:

    a. Those who ate traditional foods gave their bodies at least 10 times more of what Dr. Price called the "fat-soluble activators," or what is better known as the fat-soluble vitamins – A, D, E, and K.

    b. Those who ate traditional foods gave their bodies more essential macro-minerals calcium, phosphorus, and magnesium. They also nourished themselves with more generous amounts of essential trace minerals, such as iron and iodine.

    c. Those who ate traditional foods gave their bodies much more water-soluble

vitamins – the B complex family of nutrients and Vitamin C.

Dr. Price gradually learned a profound truth: When
people stayed faithful to their nourishing traditions, they
had little to no tooth decay or other dental problems.
He also learned that people who stayed faithful to these
traditions enjoyed significantly better overall health.

Another valuable and reciprocal part of Dr.
Price's investigations focused on what happened when
people departed from their nourishing traditions. In
all 14 cultures, when an individual or family began
to eat refined and processed foods – like white sugar,
white flour and canned food – the consequences
became evident with the onset of tooth decay. And the
longer someone ate nutrient-depleted food, the more
susceptible he or she was to developing other health
problems. Furthermore, when the children of these men
and women ate the same nutrient-depleted foods, their
incidence of tooth decay and other health problems
increased to an even higher level than their parents had.

For the rest of his life, Dr. Price faithfully taught
the lessons he had learned from his studies of nutrition:
tooth decay, crowded and/or crooked teeth, malformed
dental arches and facial bones, and even narrow nostrils
were symptoms of physical degeneration resulting from
malnutrition.

The knowledge Dr. Price gained about nutrition
eventually became a book first published in 1939 and
called *Nutrition and Physical Degeneration*. Although
some of the language is outdated, any reader interested

in nutrition will recognize that the information is of timeless value.

Included in his book are many photographs that he took of people from the cultures he studied. The comparative photos show the obvious differences in teeth and facial structure between communities that followed their nourishing traditions and those that consumed "modernized foods of commerce."

As to why Dr. Price's discoveries were not promoted to the general public, consider the potential adverse effects of his teachings on the:

✓ Sugar and sugary foods industry

✓ Soft drink industry

✓ Processed-foods industry

✓ Dental-care industry

✓ Medical-care industry

✓ Pharmaceutical industry

In 1996, a comprehensive food preparation/ cookbook based on the nutritional teachings of Dr. Price was published. It is appropriately titled *Nourishing Traditions* and was written by Sally Fallon with the help of Mary G. Enig, Ph.D. In addition to numerous recipes, the book contains valuable and practical information on nutrition. Along with Dr. Price's book, *Nutrition and Physical Degeneration*, I recommend *Nourishing Traditions, The Cookbook That Challenges Politically Correct Nutrition and the Diet Dictocrats."*

6 Steps to Getting Your Nutrition Right

Human nutrition is a complex subject. Scientists are still trying to understand all the biochemistry associated with assimilating and utilizing nutrients from our food. If that wasn't complicated enough, we now know that these processes vary from one person to another. Fortunately, your body can provide invaluable guidance.

1. Listen to Your Body

It's all too common for people to have a superficial experience with food and be aware only of the taste, texture, and temperature of what they are eating, along with a feeling of fullness in their stomach. It's possible, however, to develop some whole-body awareness of what you are eating and learn how food affects you beyond your taste buds and stomach. Your body will be one of your best nutritional advisors if you pay close attention. For most of us, life's cares and activities mute that crucial voice, but you can retrain yourself to listen and respond appropriately.

To tune in to your body's advice, start to pay attention to whether – and how – specific foods, meals, and nutritional practices affect your:

✓ Appetite

✓ Cravings

✓ Energy

✓ Mood

✓ Mental clarity

The goal is to identify foods and nutritional practices that satisfy your appetite so you don't overeat and don't have a nagging sense that "something is missing." How would you like to find the right foods and practices that

✓ Free you from cravings for sugar or anything unhealthy?

✓ Give you abundant energy?

✓ Optimize your mood?

✓ Increase your mental clarity?

Keeping a daily food diary is a valuable way to learn how you are affected by what you eat. We've included an example of a daily food diary in Appendix B. Please take a careful look at it and feel free to make copies.

As you begin to track a few bodily reactions to your eating regimen, you will start to identify and learn to avoid foods that cause you to

✓ Overeat and yet are least satisfying to your appetite

✓ Crave sugar or anything unhealthy

✓ Geel tired or even put you to sleep

✓ Have roller coaster mood swings

✓ Feel mentally dull

At a minimum, you should keep a food diary for at least a week. When the week is over, review what you have written. You will likely be amazed by what you learn from asking yourself how you feel after eating and drinking and then writing down your answers.

You will develop a nutritional intuition as you listen to your body over time. That intuition will direct you to eat natural, wholesome food perfectly suited for your body and metabolism. You will develop an inner sense that you should always trust.

2. Eat with the Intent to Nourish

When you make food choices, what is your primary intention? Is it to eat …

  A. The most nourishing food available to me and that I can afford?

  B. What tastes best?

  C. What is most convenient?

  D. As cheaply as possible?

  E. A combination of B, C, and D?

We've asked lots of people this question. Most will answer each question with "sometimes" or "it depends." Regardless of how you respond, doesn't it make sense that the best answer is "the most nourishing food available to me and I can afford"? Getting your nutrition right depends on a resolve to nourish yourself. That needs to be your primary motivation.

Enjoying what you eat is important, too, and I support that. But it's essential to go beyond how food tastes or feels in your mouth. Over time, you can re-train your taste buds so nourishing foods are appealing. When you focus on the incredible advantages, retraining is not so difficult.

3. Develop Your Nutritional Integrity

We all have standards in various areas of our life. Perhaps it involves the cleanliness of the dishes you'll eat from, how your hair looks before you venture into the public, or what grade of gas you put into your car. To get your nutrition right, you must set standards for acceptable foods and drinks for your body and stay faithful to your standards. An example of a nutritional standard would be to avoid any food with added sugar or other sweeteners.

We strongly recommend that you avoid adding sugar, "natural" sweeteners, or artificial sweeteners because these substances cause metabolic stress for your body. Additionally, the desire to use them does not result from the intention to nourish or the goal of developing nutritional integrity. There is also no doubt that "exciting" your taste buds with a concentration of sweet flavor can develop into an addictive and damaging habit.

4. Consider Your Food's Quality

A commitment to eating more wholesome food and less refined and processed food develops naturally when you are guided by the intention to nourish and the goal of nutritional integrity. Eating wholesome food containing many naturally occurring vitamins and minerals is fundamentally essential. But there is more to consider regarding the "quality of food." Making the right decisions also includes these criteria:

✓ Fresh vs. frozen

✓ Organic vs. conventional

✓ Raw vs. cooked

FRESH VS. FROZEN

There can be a significant difference between fresh and frozen food regarding nutrition and health. For some people, the difference is noticeable; for others, it isn't. But after many years of observation, I believe eating fresh food is healthier than frozen food. Frozen food still has value, but fresh food has more nutrition.

You may have noticed how frozen food, especially vegetables, fruits, and meats, can change the texture and taste. After thawing, there is some degree of "mushiness" to the texture of the food, and anywhere from a subtle to a significant loss of flavor occurs. You may have also noticed that a puddle forms around thawed-out food. This puddle is water leaking out of the cells that make up the food. It demonstrates that the cells have been damaged during the freezing process. Additionally, the water seeping from the melting food often contains essential nutrients that have leached out of the food.

How much difference does it make whether you eat fresh or frozen? There's only one way to find out. For one month, eat only fresh foods and track your energy level. Of course, locally grown food is likely to be the freshest food – and the highest in naturally occurring vitamins – so that's what I recommend whenever they are available. At the end of that time, you'll know how much of a difference it makes.

ORGANIC VS. CONVENTIONAL

Organic foods, or even better, biodynamic, perma-cultured, or wild foods (whenever available and afford-able), will have more nutritional value and flavor than conventional/factory-farmed foods. This is primarily because they are grown in better-quality soil and are not doused with agrochemicals, but let's not forget that these foods are also grown by people with a higher degree of integrity, together with a deeper apprecia-tion of the connection between the food we eat and the health we enjoy.

Besides growing it or raising your food, you should consider connecting directly with farmers whenever possible. One way to do this is to visit your area's farmers' markets. As you buy their locally grown fresh foods, talk to the farmers. Find out about their farming practices and make the most of any organic, biody-namic, permacultured, or wild foods they have available.

We also recommend shopping at stores committed to carrying reliably organic food, connecting with community-supported agriculture (CSA) programs, and joining raw dairy-based food co-ops. Raw dairy products from healthy, pasture-raised animals can be valuable for your dental and overall health. Dairy-based food co-ops usually have other high-quality foods besides raw dairy products. To find the nearest resource for raw dairy products in your area, check out realmilk.com.

Another helpful website is farmmatch.com. This website can help you find a direct-from-the-farm resource in your area. The categories you can search for are vegetables, fruits, meats, fish/seafood, dairy, eggs, grains/legumes, herbs/spices, nuts/seeds, mushrooms, and bee products. Whether you are looking for organic asparagus, zucchini, steaks, or raw butter from grass-fed animals – or any other "real" food – farmmatch.com is worth checking out.

RAW VS. COOKED

I'm not suggesting that cooked food has no nutritional value. However, depending on the type of food, there can be a significant difference. For some individuals, the difference can be subtle, and for others, the difference can be huge.

Raw foods are foods that have not been structurally altered by heat. This alteration isn't limited to plant-derived foods (vegetables, fruits, nuts, seeds, and sprouts). Animal-derived foods – eggs, dairy, seafood, and meats – are also altered by cooking. Perhaps the idea of raw meats, seafood, eggs, and dairy makes you nervous and queasy. Although this nutritional concept may be new, nourishing traditions worldwide involve eating raw-animal-derived foods. Perhaps you have even consumed some raw foods like sushi and sashimi, steak tartare, carpaccio, and kibbeh nayyeh.

Cooking food (including pasteurizing) always alters it. Different foods are affected in different ways – ranging from mild to drastic – and not all of those effects are detrimental. Besides using temperatures to "sterilize" food, cooking can make certain foods more digestible and more pleasant to consume. But cooking also reduces the nutritional value of food, making some foods less digestible and sometimes causing toxins to form. The degree and type of change depend on how much they have been cooked.

Practically speaking, experience has taught us that most people do well eating raw foods and cooked foods. There isn't one way that's right for everybody all the time – that's one of the dynamics of human nutrition in which listening to your body is indispensable. But because most people have more experience with cooked food, I have encouraged people to try raw food to see if the nutrition from raw products has more value for them. For some people, eating all or almost all their food raw is a successful way of enhancing their health. I cannot say that about people who eat all, or nearly all, of their food cooked.

There is no doubt, however, that cooked food is more attractive to the vast majority of people who want it as the basis of their diet. If you are in that group, there is some middle ground. By changing your cooking methods, structural and nutritional changes can be limited by preventing over-exposure to heat. This can be accomplished by controlling the cooking method, temperature, and cooking time. I discuss that more in the section below titled "Tips for Cooking Food."

Raw Food Tips

If you want to try raw, animal-derived foods, the book *Nourishing Traditions* can help get you started. If you want additional information, I suggest the books *We Want to Live* and *The Recipe for Living Without Disease* by Aajonus Vonderplanitz, a raw-food nutritionist. While I don't agree with everything he says (especially his recommendations on the liberal use of raw honey), these books are valuable resources.

Try eating raw-plant-derived or raw-animal-derived foods at room temperature instead of right out of the refrigerator. You may notice that they "feel" better and even taste better.

Look for organic eggs, dairy, and meat products from healthy pasture-raised animals allowed to eat the foods they instinctively seek. (This applies whether you're eating these foods raw or cooked, but especially if you're eating them raw.)

When choosing seafood, especially if consumed raw, the fresher the better, and I recommend wild, ocean-caught seafood over farm-raised seafood. Also, I strongly recommend that you avoid larger, longer-living fish like swordfish and tuna because of high levels of mercury contamination. It is generally believed that the larger the fish and the longer it lives, the more mercury (and potentially other toxic substances) it will accumulate in its body.

Tips for Cooking Food

When cooking, consider the best food preparation methods. I recommend low-temperature cooking whenever possible. Rather than using the commonly recommended – and very high – temperature of 350°F – I suggest using 225°F. Since 225°F is above the water's boiling point, 212°F, you can adequately cook any food at this temperature. The food will take longer to cook, but it won't take that much longer, and we're confident you will appreciate that the rewards are worth the longer cooking time.

Oven-Cooking Method: This method of low-temperature cooking will conserve more of the naturally occurring moisture and flavor in your food – it will taste better – and as long as you don't leave your food in the oven too long, it won't stick to the glass cookware. Most importantly, you will probably notice that your food "feels" easier to digest and is more nutritious, so you don't have to eat as much. Here's how:

✓ Use a glass casserole dish with a cover. The cover is critical. The tighter the cover fits, the better. The size of the casserole dish shouldn't be much larger than the food to be cooked.

✓ Put your food in an oven preheated to 225°F.

✓ Increase your cooking times by 50 percent from whatever they would have been at 350°F. Example: If you typically cook something at 350°F for 60 minutes, it will take about 90 minutes at 225°F.

Other Cooking Methods: Consider steaming, slow cooking (or crock pot cooking), and low-heat stovetop cooking (cooking on a simmer). These are most conducive to promoting good health.

5. Eat in Harmony with Your Metabolism

Humans share many traits and features in common. But in several ways, we are very different. We have unique fingerprints, retina patterns, and other features that start with our DNA. One area that is much less known is that we also differ in how our bodies process macronutrients – carbohydrates, proteins, and fats. Although it is critical that you get micronutrients, such as vitamins, minerals, amino acids, phytonutrients, etc., the energy essential to every bodily function comes from the macronutrients you consume.

For various reasons, some people have a metabolism that is considerably more efficient at deriving energy from carbohydrates (1), while some are much more efficient at metabolizing proteins and fats (5). We could easily represent this graphically.

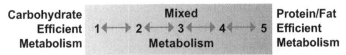

Carbohydrate Efficient Metabolism	Mixed Metabolism	Protein/Fat Efficient Metabolism
1 ◄──► 2 ◄──► 3 ◄──► 4 ◄──► 5		

A person with a carbohydrate-efficient metabolism (1) will function much better with a diet of fruits and vegetables. In contrast, someone with a protein/fat-efficient metabolism (5) will perform much better when eating animal protein and fats. Another group of people would find themselves in the middle (3). I call that a mixed metabolism. Most people have a mixed metabolism but lean closer to one side of the spectrum. I call mixed metabolisms that are more efficient with more calories derived from carbs "mixed-leaning-carb" and those who perform better on a higher level of proteins/fats "mixed-leaning-protein/fats."

Eating in harmony with your metabolism means providing a ratio of carbohydrates to proteins/fat that matches your body's metabolic disposition. The benefits of eating in this manner are significant and will positively influence your appetite, cravings, energy, mood, and mental clarity. This is an essential part of getting your nutrition right, and the first step is identifying where you are on the metabolism spectrum.

The efficiency of a person's metabolism is affected by the quality and quantity of carbohydrates, fats, and proteins and the quality and quantity of vitamins, minerals, and other nutrients in the diet. These variations in metabolism critically affect people's nutritional needs, so **there is no such thing as a diet that is good for everyone**. Additionally, After several decades of experience with thousands of people, I have learned that there isn't even one food that works well for everyone.

Low-fat vegetarian diets satisfy those on the left end of the spectrum (1). The Ornish Diet is one example. Low-carb, meat- and seafood-based diets (including eggs and some dairy products) are best for those on the right side of the spectrum (5). The Atkins Diet is an example of this approach. A few diets suggest a relatively more balanced ratio of carbohydrate, protein, and fat calories.

However, The Zone Diet and potentially the Paleo Diet are two examples.

The large segment of the population who reside on the protein/fat side of the spectrum consistently under-consumes fats and protein and over-consumes carbohydrates. These people often crave more protein and fats but suppress their intuition because they believe the false "fats-are-bad" narrative. These people also tend to be overweight or obese. They are also more prone to develop tooth decay and other dental problems.

Less often, but not uncommon, are those on the carbo metabolism side of the spectrum who are suppressing an intuition to eat fruits and grains because they have been convinced these foods are too high in carbohydrates and are trying to follow a low-carb diet. As in the previous case, these people are not healthy!

Wherever you reside on the metabolism spectrum, I recommend you trust your "nutritional intuition." Experience has taught us that almost everyone will naturally gravitate toward eating in harmony with their metabolism, at least to some extent, if they allow themselves to do so.

Identifying where you are on the spectrum will help you develop an optimal dietary strategy to achieve your best performance and health. This process isn't nearly as tricky as freeing yourself from ingrained nutritional dogma. Much of what you have heard and been taught is false or at least not true for you. All that is required to determine your metabolic tendency is honesty about how plant- and animal-derived foods affect your appetite, energy, moods, cravings, and mental clarity as you track responses to what you eat.

All five areas of guidance for getting your nutrition right (listen to your body, Intend to nourish, develop nutritional integrity, consider your food's quality, and eat in harmony with your metabolism) are crucial. However, eating in harmony with your metabolism may reap the most significant gains.

When your metabolism is balanced, your body produces and uses energy at a high level of efficiency. Your food will help contribute to calm energy, relaxed alertness, emotional poise, a positive mood, mental clarity, and good dental and overall health. Although this is not the only factor, it carries a huge impact.

When you eat in harmony with that preference, you will enjoy your food's maximum energy and nutrition. The concept is that simple. However, I've devoted the next chapter to this subject because applying this reality requires additional guidance.

6. Eat Consciously

Eating slowly and chewing your food thoroughly, as opposed to wolfing your food down, plays a vital role in determining how much nourishment you get from your food. When you eat consciously, you are much more likely to have good digestion, and you are much less likely to overeat. It's almost a closed circle: The better you digest your food, the more nourishment you get from it, and the more nourishment you get from your food, the better your health is!

It is worth considering that one of the reasons so many Americans experience digestive distress, heartburn, or acid reflux is that it has become common for people to eat while doing something else that demands all or almost all of their attention, such as working or driving. For many people, eating is just another one of the things they do while multi-tasking, and they often do it without even thinking about it. Ask some family or friends what they ate yesterday for evidence of that phenomenon. Frequently, they can't remember without writing it down.

Because eating is an essential and routine part of life, it is easy to take it for granted. When we do, we are vulnerable to developing habits such as eating too fast, not chewing well, and overeating because of a lack of attention to how much food we are putting into our mouths. People on the protein/fat metabolism side of the spectrum are especially susceptible to this.

Suggestions for Eating with More Awareness

Consider the act of taking nourishment into your body as something sacred. The food and drink you put into your body certainly have the potential to become part of your body. The expression "you are what you eat" is based on a biological truth.

Consider saying "grace" (in your way) before every meal. This can help calm your nervous system and remind you to pay attention to the food on your plate. Eating while relaxed is conducive to good digestion; eating while tense is not.

Eating slowly and chewing your food more thoroughly will be especially valuable if you wolf your food down or have digestive trouble. This simple practice doesn't cost you anything except your conscious attention, and it can have therapeutic value in reducing indigestion, heartburn, or acid reflux.

Conscious eating is complementary to the practice of listening to your body. And after making listening to your body our first guideline, I want to return to it as our last guideline as I end this chapter.

In Summary

Here are some reliable indicators that you are eating in harmony with your metabolism and doing better at getting your nutrition right:

✓ You feel more satisfied with what you eat and do not have a nagging sense that something is missing.

✓ You can go longer after eating before you begin to feel hungry. Also, when you feel hungry, it is more of a calm kind of hunger rather than an urgent I've-got-to-eat-something-now type of hunger. (This is especially true for people on the protein/fat metabolism side of the spectrum.)

✓ Snacking between meals or before bedtime is no longer necessary because after eating breakfast or lunch, you can go about four to six hours before you feel hungry again. After dinner, you can easily make it through the night without getting hungry.

✓ You no longer have sugar cravings or cravings for something unhealthy.

✓ Your digestion and elimination are functioning well.

✓ Your energy level is more consistent. You are not feeling tired all the time.

✓ Your mood is better. You are not on a roller-coaster.

✓ Your mental clarity is more consistent. You do not have brain fog.

✓ You feel that your health is improving.

CHAPTER 11

Eating in Harmony with Your Metabolism

The previous chapter listed six steps for getting your nutrition right. Eating in harmony with your metabolic tendency was an important one of those. This step is critical for maintaining a health-promoting terrain in your mouth and your entire body. I want to provide a more in-depth explanation for those unfamiliar with this crucial dietary concept.

Before you can eat in harmony with your metabolism, you need to know where you reside on the metabolic spectrum. If you remember, I set up the spectrum like this:

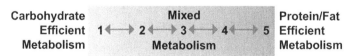

Carbohydrate Efficient Metabolism		Mixed Metabolism		Protein/Fat Efficient Metabolism
1	2	3	4	5

With the highly carbohydrate-efficient metabolism on the far left, the high protein/fat-efficient metabolism on the right, and the perfectly mixed metabolism in the middle. Those with carbo metabolism and people with protein/fat metabolism have the most distinctive characteristics.

To start the process of locating yourself on the spectrum, do the following:

✓ Carefully read through all the carbo metabolism characteristics. Take note of which ones, if any, you identify with.

✓ Carefully read through all the protein/fat metabolism characteristics and note which ones, if any, you identify with.

Carbohydrate Metabolism Characteristics

Read the characteristics below, and check all that apply:

☐ I consistently look forward to and feel good when I eat vegetables, fruits, and grains.

☐ Eating vegetables and fruits helps restore my energy, whereas meats/seafood don't seem to have that effect.

☐ Freshly made vegetable juice gives me energy, and to a lesser degree, so does fresh-squeezed fruit juice.

☐ If my eating described me, I "eat to live" rather than "live to eat."

☐ Eating a simple vegetable salad satisfies my appetite when hungry.

☐ I usually do not overeat starchy food such as

bread or potato, and I prefer to have just a tiny amount of butter or oil on these foods, if any.

☐ If I had to choose either the white or the yolk of a hard-boiled egg - I would choose the white.

☐ I usually have no interest and can even feel repulsed by liver, sardines, bacon, sausage, and other fatty meats.

☐ Over-consuming fatty and oily food is the primary dietary cause of weight gain and feeling low in energy.

☐ When overweight, a low-fat 'plant-based' diet will help me to lose weight, gain energy, and improve my overall health.

Divide the number of checked boxes in the Carbo Metabolism Characteristics by ten to determine your percent of carbo metabolism tendencies.

Protein/Fat Metabolism Characteristics

Read the characteristics below and check all that apply:

☐ I consistently look forward to and feel good about meat and seafood nutrition.

☐ I consistently look forward to and feel good when I eat meat or seafood.

☐ If I had to choose between eating meat and seafood OR vegetables and fruits to restore my energy – I would select meats and seafood.

☐ A rare, juicy steak or burger (without a bun), liver, or sardines can be especially energizing.

☐ My relationship with food could be described as 'lives to eat' rather than 'eats to live.'

☐ Eating a vegetable salad by itself will have little value in satisfying my appetite when hungry.

☐ I have a strong tendency to eat fast

☐ I love cheese and butter!

☐ If I had to choose either the yolk or the white of a hard-boiled egg – I would choose the yolk.

☐ I don't enjoy eating bread or potato unless I can have it with lots of butter or oil.

☐ I feel indifferent about most vegetables and salads, especially when hungry.

☐ A meal high in starch and/or sugar will NOT satisfy my appetite for long or at all and can leave me feeling wired but tired or sleepy.

☐ Over-consuming carbs is the primary dietary cause of gaining weight and losing energy.

☐ When overweight, a low-carb keto-type diet can help me lose weight, gain energy, and improve my overall health.

☐ A meal that starts with a serving of meat or seafood followed by a serving of low-carb vegetables with cheese and then a bit of starch with butter is very satisfying.

☐ A meal that starts with fresh vegetables and/ or fruit nutrition (especially juice and a salad) followed by some whole grain and/or yogurt or light-colored fish or white poultry meat - is not very satisfying.

Divide the number of checked boxes in the Protein/Fat Metabolism Characteristics by fifteen to determine your percent of protein/fat tendencies.

Refining Your Location on the Metabolism Spectrum

Compare your percentage of carbo metabolism tendencies with your protein/fat metabolism preferences. Although far from precise, this will indicate where you live on the Metabolism Energy Spectrum. Start there and adjust as you track your feelings in your Food Diary (see Appendix A). To summarize, there are five basic possibilities:

1.   Carbo metabolism

2.   Mixed, leaning towards carbo metabolism

3.   Mixed

4.   Mixed, leaning towards protein/fat metabolism

5.   Protein/fat metabolism

You will always have a place on the spectrum. You may shift slightly to the right or left or even change significantly because of your biological cycles or rhythms, seasonal changes, or the ebb and flow of stress you are under. Nevertheless, as long as you are alive, you will always be somewhere on the spectrum!

How Failing to Eat Harmoniously Impacts the Mouth and Teeth

To emphasize the importance of eating in harmony with your metabolism tendencies, I will give you an example of how being out of harmony impacts the terrain of your mouth. When people with protein/fat metabolism eat too many carbs and do not get enough protein/fat, they are much more vulnerable to tooth decay. Conversely, those with a carb metabolism who are not eating a sufficient quantity and quality carbohydrates are much more vulnerable to periodontal disease than tooth decay. As you might expect, when people with mixed metabolisms aren't getting their nutrition right, they are more susceptible to tooth decay and periodontal disease.

Once you have identified where you are on the metabolism spectrum, it's time to learn the basics of eating harmoniously with it. Of course, it's fundamentally important to eat real food! With this in mind, you may want to write a reminder to put on your refrigerator door or another prominent location:

The best food is simple, real food that does not have a label with a list of ingredients.

Identifying Real Food Groups

To cover all real foods in a general way, I have divided them into nine primary groups within two broad categories: plant-derived foods and animal-derived foods. (See food group charts on following pages.)

General Eating Guidelines

Identifying where you are on the spectrum can be especially valuable if you have carbo or protein/fat metabolism because they have more specific nutritional requirements than someone with a mixed metabolism. Many misconceptions exist about carbs, proteins, and fats because most people are unaware of metabolic tendencies and the spectrum. Therefore, you must avoid buying into an unbalanced dietary strategy, such as a low-fat vegan diet or a low-carb/high-protein and fat diet, as the way you "should be" eating.

My guidelines for helping you eat in harmony with your metabolism are based on the two general categories, nine primary food groups, and the subgroups identified within each basic group. The suggestions for each metabolic tendency will include primary, secondary, fine-tuning, and occasional food when appropriate, using foods from the general categories, primary food groups, and subgroups. My guidelines only include food that is a recommended part of your nutrition plan.

Due to much hype from the pharmaceutical industry, there is a high level of worry about cholesterol. I believe it's not a concern if you eat foods compat-

Plant-Derived Foods

Category	Subgroups	Comments
Vegetables The caloric value of vegetables is primarily carbohydrate, with some protein and a trace amount of fat.	**Lower-Carb Vegetables**	The vast majority of vegetables that are lower carb grow above the ground. *Examples include*: • Asparagus • Lettuce • Bell pepper • Mushrooms1 • Broccoli • Onions • Cabbage • Radicchio • Cauliflower • Radishes2 • Celery • Seaweed3 • Cucumber • Spinach • Fennel • String Beans •Greens,all leafy •Tomato 1 Although mushrooms are fungi, for practical purposes, consider them lower-carb vegetables. 2 Radishes and onions are lower-carb vegetables that grow below the ground. 3 Varieties of seaweed, such as dulse and kelp, also qualify as lower-carb vegetables.
	Higher-Carb Vegetables	The vast majority of vegetables that are higher carb grow below the ground. *Examples include:* • Artichoke • Parsnips Hearts[4] • Potatoes • Beets • Yams • Carrots • Squash[4] 4 Artichoke hearts and squash (summer and especially winter varieties) are higher-carb vegetables that grow above the ground.
Fruits The caloric value of sweet fruits is predominantly carbohydrate with a little bit of protein and a trace amount of fat. Fatty fruits contain mostly fat calories, a small to moderate amount of carbs and some protein.	**Sweet Fruits Eaten With** Peel or Skin	*Examples include*: • Apples • Pears • Apricots • Peaches • Berries • Persimmons • Cherries • Plums

	Sweet Fruits Eaten Without Peel or Skin	*Examples include*:
		• Bananas • Melons
		• Citrus • Pineapple
		   (Oranges, and other
		   Lemons, tropical fruits
		   Limes, • Pomegranate
		   Grapefruit, etc.)

	Fatty Fruits Eaten With Peel or Skin	*Examples include*: • Avocados • Olives • Coconuts

Plant-Derived Foods

Category	Subgroups	Comments
Grains All grains are high in carbs, with some protein and a small amount of fat.		*Examples include*: • Oats • spelt • wild rice • barley • brown rice • corn • quinoa • wheat • millet • rye
Legumes For the vast majority the caloric value is primarily carbohydrate, with a significant amount of protein and at least a little bit of fat. In general, legumes are somewhat lower in carbs and somewhat higher in protein than grains. A few legumes, most notably soybeans, have a more moderate carbohydrate value with a higher amount of protein and fat.		*Examples include*: • Oats • spelt • wild rice • barley • brown rice • corn • quinoa • wheat • millet • rye
Nuts and Seeds The caloric value of nuts and seeds is predominantly fat calories, along with some protein and carbohydrate value.		*Examples include*: **Nuts** **Seeds** • Almonds • Chia • Brazil Nuts • Flax • Cashews[5] • Hemp • Peanuts[5] • Pumpkin • Pecans • Sesame • Pistachios • Sunflower • Walnuts 6 Although peanuts and cashews are officially legumes, for practical purposes consider them nuts.

Animal-Derived Foods

Category	Subgroups	Comments
Meat In general, the caloric value of meat is predominantly protein with some fat or predominantly fat with some protein but with at least a trace amount of carbohydrate.	**Red Meat**	Beef, bison, lamb, venison
	Poultry Dark Meat	The leg and thigh
	Poultry White Meat	Breast and wing
	Pork, Wild Game, Organ Meats	Liver, heart, kidney etc.
Seafood Generally, the caloric value of seafood is predominantly protein with some fat or predominantly fat with some protein but with at least a trace amount of carbohydrate.	**Light-Colored**	Sole, cod, haddock, etc.
	Darker-Colored Fish	Salmon, sardines, arctic char, etc.
	Shellfish	Shrimp, oysters, scallops, etc. and Roe (fish eggs)
	Pork, Wild Game, Organ Meats	Liver, heart, kidney etc.
Dairy Whole milk (from which all the other dairy products are derived) is mostly fat calories, together with substantial amounts of carbohydrate and protein calories.	**Milk, kefir and yogurt**	Dairy products with the highest carbohydrate value
	Butter, cheese, cream and cottage cheese	Dairy products with no to low carbohydrate value
Eggs	**Chicken and Duck**	A whole egg consists of mostly fat calories, with a substantial amount of protein and a bit of carbohydrate. All of the fat nutrition in an egg is in the yolk

ible with where you are on the spectrum for nutrient metabolism.

> **IMPORTANT:**
> With all of my recommendations, be sure to exclude any foods to which you have an allergy or intolerance.

What is a Primary Food?

Primary foods are essential for a balanced metabolism. You will want to eat these every day and at every meal. Your meal plan should begin with choosing your primary food as defined under each metabolism tendency. I also recommend eating your primary foods as the first part of a meal. This can be invaluable in achieving a more balanced metabolism. It can help satisfy your nutritional and energy needs more efficiently while lengthening the time before you feel hungry again. For many people, this practice provides an immediate benefit. Try it for a while and monitor how you feel.

What is a Secondary Food?

Secondary food is necessary for balanced metabolism but complementary to primary food. It is everyday food but not necessarily every-meal food. Try having secondary food after starting a meal with primary food, but then feel free to have more primary food (especially vegetable or fruit nutrition) with your secondary food. Remember, primary food is every day, every-meal food and is needed to create a complete meal.

What is an Occasional Food?

Occasional foods are not required! You don't have to eat occasional food for a balanced metabolism, but it can still be valuable. If you want occasional food, I recommend doing so a few times a week and keeping your servings small.

What is Fine-Tuning Food?

A small amount of fine-tuning food may be needed to "complete" a meal for someone with a protein/fat metabolism. These people need some carbohydrates, and this food is meant to provide enough of them to support balanced metabolism. Fine-tuning food should be reserved for the end of a meal after eating the primary and secondary food. Those with a protein/fat metabolism often realize that just one mouthful of fine-tuning food is all that is needed! In small amounts, this food can be everyday food and even every-meal food.

Carbo Metabolism Eating Guidelines

General

Perhaps, in the past, you followed a plan that leaned toward vegetarian meals and provided most of your calories from good-quality carbohydrates derived primarily from vegetables, fruits, and grains. It also included nutrition from some animal-derived foods. Suppose you felt healthy and satisfied with following this plan. In that case, my advice is to trust your own experience and consider returning to this way of eating, especially if someone convinced you to stop because the diet was too high in carbs or you stopped following it for another reason.

Primary Foods for a Carbo Metabolism

Select your foods from these categories:
✓ Vegetables
✓ Fruits
✓ Grains

Special Notes: Eat your selected items first. This can help your carbo metabolism run more efficiently. Make it a priority to get the nutrition from fresh vegetables into your body every day and include some leafy greens. Citrus fruit can be especially beneficial for someone with a carbo metabolism.

Secondary Foods for a Carbo Metabolism

Food that will be complimentary to your primary foods should be selected from these categories and subgroups:
✓ Dairy
✓ Eggs
✓ Nut/Seeds
✓ Light-Colored Fish
✓ White Meat Poultry

Special Notes: Reduced-fat dairy products often feel best to people with a carbo metabolism. When consuming cooked egg nutrition, it may be best to have two or even three egg whites for each egg yolk. Nut and seed nutrition can be most valuable when whole, raw nuts or seeds are soaked in water for eight to 24 hours before consumption.

Occasional Foods for a Carbo Metabolism

Foods that can be added a few times per week (less than one serving per day) should be selected from these categories and subgroups:

✓ Cheese
✓ Fatty fruits
✓ Legumes

Special Notes: If you make fresh juice, mix mainly lower-carb vegetables and some higher-carb vegetables and fruit. For a blended smoothie, feel free to use fewer lower-carb vegetables and more higher-carb vegetables and fruit.

Protein/Fat Metabolism Eating Guidelines

General

If you followed a "low-carb" plan that consisted of good-quality, animal-derived fat and protein and also included a good amount of vegetables, but you stopped following this plan because someone convinced you it was too high in fat or protein and that it would not be good for your long-term health, or you stopped following it for some other reason even though you felt well while following it, my advice is to trust your own experience and consider going back to the nutrition plan that was enhancing your health.

People with protein/fat metabolism who are not eating enough of the right meat or seafood will often have a nagging sense that something is missing from their nutrition. They also may describe themselves as feeling hungry all the time or almost all the time. The practice of eating enough of the right kind of meat or seafood to start a meal often has a dramatic effect on completely satisfying their appetite.

At any meal, when people with protein/fat metabolism eat meat or seafood first – before consuming any other food – they may not need much. For some people, a serving as small as a couple of ounces feels just right, but a more substantial quantity is required for most people with protein/fat metabolism. Listen to your body and allow it to guide you.

A person with a protein/fat metabolism usually needs to eat meat or seafood at least twice daily. A meal starting with a serving of red meat, dark-meat poultry, pork, shellfish, or darker-colored, oily fish like salmon, followed by a serving of low-carb vegetables with cheese and then a tiny starch portion with butter, will feel very satisfying.

Primary Foods for a Protein/Fat Metabolism

Select your foods from these categories and subgroups:

✓ Meat
✓ Seafood – darker-colored, oily fish; shellfish; and roe (fish eggs)

Special Notes: For starters, try this meal-plan strategy: Have a serving of meat or seafood first and finish it before you have any other food. Pay attention to how this affects satisfying your appetite and meeting your energy needs. Getting nutrition from meat or seafood before consuming other foods can help your protein/fat metabolism run more efficiently. Prioritize buying the best quality meat and seafood you can afford. Consuming a variety of meats and seafood can help you get a better balance of essential nutrients, especially minerals.

If your appetite is relatively light, cheese and/or eggs – duck eggs more so than chicken eggs – may be nutritionally satisfying substitutes for meat or seafood. If you have a normal to hefty appetite, consider cheese and eggs exclusively as secondary food.

Sometimes the white meat of poultry and light-colored fish is not as satisfying for someone with a protein/fat metabolism. If that is true of you, leave them off your meal plan. However, if they satisfy you to some extent, please include them, along with your primary meat or seafood.

Secondary Foods for a Protein/Fat Metabolism

Food that will be complimentary to your primary foods should be selected from these subgroups:

✓ **Lower-Carb Vegetables** – Specific lower-carb vegetables that can be most valuable for someone with protein/fat metabolism are asparagus, spinach, mushrooms, cauliflower, celery, artichoke leaves, string beans, and kelp. Feel free to include any other lower-carb vegetables that appeal to you.

✓ Dairy

✓ Eggs

✓ Nuts and Seeds

✓ Fatty Fruits

We suggest eating your secondary food only after finishing your primary food. Make it a priority to have some lower-carb vegetables in combination with butter, cheese, cottage cheese, cream, egg, nut, seed, or fatty fruit.

Fine-Tuning Foods for a Protein/Fat Metabolism

Fine-tuning food, in small amounts, can be everyday food or even every-meal food. Feel free to have more secondary food, such as butter, cream, or cheese, with fine-tuning food.
   ✓ Higher-Carb Vegetables
   ✓ Legumes
   ✓ Dairy

Occasional Fine-Tuning Foods for a Protein/Fat Metabolism

These fine-tuning foods from once to no more than several times a week may help satisfy some of your nutrition needs. Feel free to have more secondary food, such as butter, nuts, or seeds, with these foods.
   ✓ Sweet fruits, eaten with their peel or skin
   ✓ Grains – See caution below
   Grain Caution: Some people should avoid including grains in their meal plans. For many with protein/fat metabolism, grains are a food group they are prone to overeating. To prevent over-eating, follow my guidelines for fine-tuning food and reserve any grain for the end of a meal after you have had primary and secondary food. If you do this and are satisfied with a small serving of grain, include it in your weekly meal

plan as an occasional fine-tuning food. If, however, having a little grain causes you to want a lot more, I recommend keeping grains off your meal plan.

You need to understand that you must be careful with carbohydrates! If you are not consuming enough protein and fat, you will inevitably over-consume carbohydrates, which can hurt your dental and overall health.

Mixed Metabolism Eating Guidelines

General

If you have a mixed metabolism, are unhappy with your food or health, or are drawn toward eating various plant- and animal-derived foods, try implementing a mixed-metabolism nutrition plan. On the other hand, if you are satisfied with your nutrition and health, stick with what works for you.

Primary Foods for a Mixed Metabolism

Select your foods from these categories:
✓ Lower-Carb Vegetables
✓ Eggs
✓ Dairy
✓ Seafood
✓ Meat

Secondary Foods for a Mixed Metabolism

At least for a week or so, try having secondary food after consuming primary food. If you want to try a small amount of secondary food with your primary food, feel free to do so. However, consider whether this practice is more effective in satisfying your appetite and providing energy. Food that will be complimentary to your primary foods should be selected from these subgroups:

✓ Higher-Carb Vegetables
✓ Fruits
✓ Nuts and Seeds
✓ Legumes
✓ Grains
✓ Dairy – cream and butter

Familiar combinations include a salad with some protein/fat added – an egg salad, a chicken salad, or another meat salad – and vegetable soup. Stews, or chili with added meat or seafood, are all in harmony with the nutritional needs of someone with a mixed metabolism.

Mixed-Leaning-Protein/Fat Metabolism Eating Guidelines

General

Plant-derived foods should be favored over animal-derived foods for people with mixed leaning toward a carbo metabolism. Most of your calories should come from carbohydrates but only a little more than protein or fat. Consuming a variety of plant- and animal-derived food is highly recommended.

Primary Foods for a Mixed-Leaning-Carbo Metabolism

Try starting a meal with a small (appetizer-size) serving of vegetable or fruit and then follow it with one of these alternatives:

✓ Another serving of vegetable or fruit
   nutrition, combined with dairy or egg
✓ Some vegetables with fish or poultry
✓ A serving of milk, kefir, or yogurt

Select your primary foods from these categories:

✓ Vegetables – A mix of mostly lower-
   carb and some higher-carb vegetables is
   recommended.
✓ Fruits
✓ Dairy
✓ Eggs – chicken
✓ Light-Colored Fish
✓ White Meat of Poultry

Secondary Foods for a Mixed-Leaning-Carbo Metabolism

At least for a week or so, try having secondary food after consuming primary food. If you want to try a small amount of secondary food with your primary food, feel free to do so. However, consider whether this practice is more effective in satisfying your appetite and providing energy. Feel free to have secondary food at every meal, but also feel free to skip secondary food at any meal.

Select your secondary foods from this list of categories and subgroups:

✓   •   Grains
✓   •   Legumes
✓   •   Nuts and Seeds
✓   •   Fatty Fruits
✓   •   Dairy – cream and butter

Occasional Foods for a Mixed-Leaning-Carbo Metabolism

You may need occasional food once a week or so to help satisfy some of your nutritional needs and help you maintain a balanced metabolism. Have some primary food first (especially vegetables) before having occasional food. Select your occasional foods from these categories:

✓ Seafood – darker-colored fish, shellfish, and roe
✓ Meat – dark meat of poultry, red meat, organ meats, wild game, and pork

Mixed-Leaning-Protein/Fat Metabolism Eating Guidelines

General

For people with mixed leaning toward protein/fat metabolism, animal-derived foods should be favored, to some degree, over plant-derived foods. Consuming more calories from protein and fat (but not too much more) than from carbohydrates will help your metabolism run more efficiently. However, it's best to eat a variety of plant- and animal-derived food.

Primary Foods for a Mixed-Leaning-Protein/Fat Metabolism

As a starting point, follow a meal plan based on having meat, seafood, eggs, or dairy before or with lower-carb vegetables. Try eating primary foods first at each main meal. The hungrier you are, the more critical it is to eat some, or even all, of your primary protein and fat first, but don't overlook at least a small amount of secondary food. Remember, primary food is essential in maintaining a balanced metabolism, so creating a meal plan should begin with choosing primary food. Select your secondary foods from these categories:

✓ Meat
✓ Seafood
✓ Eggs
✓ Dairy – cheese and cottage cheese
✓ Lower-Carb Vegetables

Secondary Foods for a Mixed-Leaning-Protein/Fat Metabolism

Try having secondary food after finishing your primary food. It would be best if you had secondary food to have a balanced metabolism but complementary to primary food. Remember to include secondary food daily as it is required to create a "complete" meal. Have at least a small serving of secondary food with every main meal.

You may select your secondary foods from this list of categories and subgroups:

✓ Higher-Carb Vegetables
✓ Dairy – butter, cream, milk, kefir, and yogurt
✓ Nuts and Seeds
✓ Sweet Fruits – those eaten with the peel or skin
✓ Fatty Fruits
✓ Legumes

Occasional Foods for a Mixed-Leaning-Protein/Fat Metabolism

You don't need occasional food for a balanced metabolism, but it can still be valuable. If you're interested in having occasional food, I recommend doing so no more than several times a week and keeping your serving size small.

Select your occasional foods from this list of categories and subgroups:

✓ Grains
✓ Sweet Fruits – those eaten without the peel or skin

In Summary

If you don't get your assessment right at first and follow the wrong guidelines, you won't receive any benefits, and you may experience an increase in cravings, a decrease in energy, or a sense that "this isn't right for me." But the good news is that you're much more likely to get your assessment right on the next try!

We all experience the ebb and flow of life, and it is to be expected that we will also experience some dynamics in the activity of our metabolism. When your metabolism changes, so will your nutritional needs. No matter where you are on the spectrum, rather than thinking of your metabolism as a type, I recommend that you think of it as your tendency, which implies some movement in your metabolism. Because of this, you need to listen to your body and trust your nutritional intuition.

Proper nutrition is a lifelong responsibility and an exciting adventure. If you are interested in a holistic approach to your health, you realize that nutrition plays a significant role in the maintenance and well-being of your body. You know proper nutrition is crucial for your heart, liver, lungs, and kidneys. But It's just as essential for your teeth and other structures in your mouth.

Human nutrition is a complex subject. Scientists are still trying to understand all the biochemistry associated with assimilating and utilizing nutrients from our food. If that wasn't complicated enough, we now know that these processes vary from one person to another. Fortunately, your body can provide invaluable guidance.

CHAPTER 12

Fluoride is Not Your Friend?

Introduction: What is Fluoride?

"Fluoride" is a generic term describing a chemical compound containing fluorine and one or more additional elements. In its pure state, fluorine is a yellowish gas that is highly corrosive and poisonous. It is known to be the most reactive of all the non-metallic elements in the Periodic Table of Elements. Because of this, fluorine exists in nature only in combination with at least one other element. So, fluorine + calcium = calcium fluoride; fluorine + sodium + aluminum = sodium aluminum fluoride.

Significant amounts of fluoride occur naturally in the Earth's crust. In contrast, fluoride occurs in trace amounts in the oceans, and in most fresh-water sources, fluoride is often found at just a fraction of the trace amount found in oceans.

Because of the prevalence of fluoride in the Earth's crust, industries that mine for raw materials inevitably produce varying amounts of fluoride-containing hazardous waste as a byproduct of their extraction and refinement processes. Fluorides are the primary waste products of several enterprises, such as the phosphate fertilizer and aluminum industries.

What Is Water Fluoridation?

The American Dental Association (ADA) states that water fluoridation is "The ADA recognizes the use of fluoride and community water fluoridation as safe and effective in preventing tooth decay for both children and adults"[1] and the Centers for Disease Control and Prevention (CDC) refer to water fluoridation as "one of 10 great public health achievements of the 20th century."[2]

A concise, no-nonsense way of describing what water fluoridation amounts to is this: Local governments spend tax dollars to buy fluoride-rich hazardous waste, primarily from the phosphate fertilizer industry, and dump it into our water supplies because it's supposed to be good for our teeth.

Let's evaluate these statements in order.

Is Fluoride Safe?

Fluoride naturally occurs in the phosphate-rich rocks that are used to make fertilizer. Fertilizer manu-

---

1. https://www.ada.org/-/media/project/a2da-organization/ada/ ada-org/files/community-initiatives/fluoridation_statements_ from_leading_authorities.pdf
2. https://blogs.cdc.gov/pcd/2015/04/23/community-water-fluo- ridation-one-of-the-10-greatest-public-health-achievements-of- the-20th-century

facturers treat these rocks with sulfuric acid to free the phosphate compounds from the mined rocks. This procedure releases two highly toxic gases: hydrogen fluoride and silicon tetrafluoride. The Environmental Protection Agency (EPA) has classified these byproducts as environmental pollutants and hazardous waste. It requires factories to capture these gases because they are known to damage crops, injure animals, and harm humans.

To prevent the release of hydrogen fluoride and silicon tetrafluoride, fertilizer plants use smokestack scrubbers that spray these toxic gases with water. This process produces a new compound, hydrofluorosilicic acid (hexafluorosilicic acid or fluorosilicic acid). The resulting wastewater that accumulates also contains arsenic and other toxic byproducts from the phosphate-rich rocks. Rather than go to great expense to properly dispose of hydrofluorosilicic acid as hazardous waste, it is loaded into tanker trucks and sold to municipalities nationwide. These cities then dump this toxic acid into their water supplies – supposing their "fluoride treatment" will help prevent cavities in those who drink the city's water.

In a 1983 letter written by Deputy Assistant Administrator for Water at the EPA, Rebecca Hanmer said, "In regard to the use of fluorosilicic acid as a source of fluoride for fluoridation, this agency regards such use as an ideal environmental solution to a long-standing problem. By recovering by-product fluorosilicic acid from fertilizer manufacturing, **water and air pollu-**

tion are minimized, and water utilities have a low-cost source of fluoride available to them."[3] (emphasis added)

Even though fluoridated water is considered "safe to drink," you only need to look at any tube of fluoride-containing toothpaste to find the following warning: "If more than used for brushing is accidentally swallowed, *get medical help or contact a Poison Control Center right away.*" (emphasis added)

Much more troubling is the recent finding of a 6-year systematic review of fluoride's impact on the developing brain conducted by the National Toxicology Program (NTP). This program is part of the U.S. Department of Health and Human Services (HHS). The program's report states that 52 of 55 studies found decreases in child IQ associated with increased fluoride. It reported that:

> "Our meta-analysis confirms results of previous meta-analyses and extends them by including newer, more precise studies with individual-level exposure measures. The data support a consistent inverse association between fluoride exposure and children's IQ."[4]

A meta-analysis combines data from all relevant studies, which is then statistically analyzed to produce a fuller, unbiased overall picture. The NTP's meta-analysis also put the magnitude of harm into perspective:

---

3. https://fluoridealert.org/news/
   lawmakers-should-vote-to-stop-fluoridation/

4. https://fluoridealert.org/articles/national-toxicology-pro-
   gram-finds-no-safe-level-of-fluoride-in-drinking-water-wa-
   ter-fluoridation-policy-threatened/

"[R]esearch on other neurotoxicants has shown that subtle shifts in IQ at the population level can profoundly impact the number of people who fall within the high and low ranges of the population's IQ distribution. For example, a 5-point decrease in a population's IQ would nearly **double that of people classified as intellectually disabled.**" (emphasis added)

An average drop of 5 IQ points in a population might sound small, but it is enormous from a public health perspective – doubling the number of disabled persons is massive! But even more sobering, the report stated there was the potential for some people to be more susceptible than average. These sensitive individuals could lose 10, 15, 20, or more IQ points, which would likely cause profound lifetime negative consequences.

Even though all five independent peer-reviewers of the NTP report voted to accept the review's main conclusion and lauded the report, the HHS leadership blocked and concealed the information from the public for ten months until a court ruled that it be released.

The World Health Organization (WHO) recommends that a maximum level of 1.5 mg/L of fluoride be added to drinking water to remain safe, and the level considered optimal in the United States is 0.7 mg/L. Even so, In numerous responses to comments by reviewers of the report, the NTP made clear that they had found evidence that exposures of at least some people in areas with these "optimal" levels were associated with lower child IQ. The NTP report stated:

"Several of the highest quality studies showing lower IQs in children were done in optimally fluoridated (0.7 mg/L) areas...many urinary fluoride measurements exceed those that would be expected from consuming water that contains fluoride at 1.5 mg/L."[5]

A research program within the United States government shows severe neurotoxicity due to fluoride exposures below what is considered safe. Yet, as of this writing, hazardous fluoride waste is being dumped into municipal drinking water nationwide.

But there's more to this intentional fluoride exposure. First, no government agency is responsible for monitoring the effects of fluoridated water on any organ, gland, or body system other than teeth. (This applies, as well, to the ADA or any other professional association.) Medical science is well aware that, throughout our lives, fluoride accumulates in our bones. It is reasonable to consider that this can lead to joint trouble. Considering all the people in the U.S. who have arthritis, it is essential to know that chronic fluoride toxicity can cause symptoms similar to arthritis.

Fluoride impacts other parts of the body as well. For many years, fluoride has been used to treat people with hyperthyroidism because it has proven to be a very effective drug for decreasing thyroid gland activity. Even now, fluoridated water and other products might adversely affect many U.S. people challenged with hypo-

_____

5. https://fluoridealert.org/articles/national-toxicology-program-
   finds-no-safe-level-of-fluoride-in-drinking-water-water-
   fluoridation-policy-threatened/

thyroidism (a condition in which insufficient thyroid hormone is produced).

If you want to know more about the dangers of water fluoridation, I highly recommend *The Case Against Fluoride*. This book, published in 2010, has extensive information about water fluoridation's history, economics, and politics. The book's subtitle is also quite telling: *How Hazardous Waste Ended Up in Our Drinking Water, and the Bad Science and Powerful Politics That Keep It There.*

The politics are alarming! Until the tanker trucks loaded with fluorosilicic acid deliver it to the water-fluoridating municipalities, it's considered hazardous material – and then, in some unknown and apparently "magical" way, it instantly becomes suitable for human consumption!

Ingesting fluoridated water is likely to result in other health problems because fluoride can inhibit enzyme activity, interfere with the body's utilization of the essential nutrients calcium and iodine, and increase the stress from free radicals, which are highly reactive and unstable molecules, on cells throughout the body. Fluoride's effects on the biochemistry of the human body are antagonistic to good health.

When investigating the scientific research that examines how fluoride can affect our body (beyond our teeth), we learn that fluoride accumulates, especially in our bones, but also in other areas, such as the pineal gland, which is linked to our sleep cycle, among other things. Fluoride can also increase our risk for numerous health problems, including gastrointestinal irritation, skin rashes, symptoms similar to arthritis, hypothyroidism (insufficient thyroid production), and kidney damage.

Is Fluoride Beneficial and Cost-Effective for Preventing Dental Caries

"It is essential that in considering the dental caries problem, it shall be kept in mind ... that it is only one of a large group of symptoms of modern physical degeneration, and when teeth are decaying, other things are going wrong in the body. Fluorine (fluoride) treatment, like dental extractions, cannot be a panacea for dental caries." – Dr. Weston A. Price, 1945

Dental decay is a symptom of a disruption of the body's terrain. The toxicity of fluoride can only further disrupt it, causing, or at least exacerbating, some of the dysfunction in the body already. Consider these facts:

✓ Fluoride has no nutritional value for any structure in the body, including the teeth. Therefore, tooth decay does not occur because of a fluoride deficiency, nor is fluoride necessary for the prevention of tooth decay.

✓ Although when topically applied to teeth, fluoride can have a superficial effect on reducing cavities in many people, that same effect is not observed when people consume fluoridated water.

✓ Ingesting too much fluoride can harm children's teeth, as fluoride is the causative factor for an injury known as dental fluorosis.

Fluorosis is a condition in which the enamel of the teeth is damaged by over-exposure to fluoride while teeth are developing.

Data from the CDC confirms that 1 out of 3 children in the U.S. between the ages of 6 and 11 and 2 out of 5 children between the ages of 12 and 15 have some degree of dental fluorosis.[6] In mild cases, the abnormal changes in the enamel can appear as small white spots or streaks. Still, in severe cases, the enamel becomes discolored with brown spots, along with significant pitting and markedly increased brittleness of the teeth. The politically correct way of explaining dental fluorosis is to say a child has been "overexposed" to fluoride. But an honest and no-nonsense way of explaining dental fluorosis is this: It is a physical symptom that a child has experienced some degree of chronic fluoride poisoning.

From a scientific and holistic perspective, it doesn't make sense to support the fluoridation of our water supplies, especially when we don't even need fluoride to prevent cavities. A deficiency of fluoride does not cause cavities. Fluoride is a toxin – not a nutrient. Cavities are primarily caused by poor nutrition – especially eating more sugar than our body can handle – and inadequate oral hygiene.

---

6. https://www.cdc.gov/nchs/products/databriefs/db53.htm

How Did Water Fluoridation Become the National Norm?

Our government first began to promote water fluoridation in the 1950s. Edward Bernays was one of the men called upon to help sell the idea to the American people. He had just written a book called *Propaganda*. His book is an excellent example of its subject in action. Not only did the book try to justify the use of propaganda, but it tried to glorify it.

Bernays was considered highly accomplished in the "engineering of consent" business and wrote a book with the same name. For instance, Bernays wrote,

> "If we understand the mechanism and motives of the group mind, is it not possible to control and regiment the masses according to our will without them knowing about it? The recent practice of propaganda has proved that it is possible, at least up to a certain point and within certain limits."[7]

Fluoridation of water was not his only success story. He is called "the father of public relations," as he devised a successful propaganda campaign that persuaded many American women to start smoking cigarettes in the 1920s.

> "After WWI, Bernays was hired by the American Tobacco Company to encourage women to start smoking. While men smoked cigarettes, it was not publicly acceptable for women to smoke. Bernays staged a dramatic public display of women smoking during the Easter Day Parade in New York City. He then told the press to expect that women suffragists would

---

7. http://pr.wikia.com/wiki/Edward_Bernays

light up "torches of freedom" during the parade to show they were equal to men."[8]

It's now apparent that the government's and ADA's promotion of water fluoridation as "a safe, beneficial and cost-effective, public-health measure for preventing dental caries" was and is propaganda, not science.

Why Are Cities Still Fluoridating Their Water?

The short answer is ignorance and apathy. These are the allies of fluoridation promoters, who rely on the reluctance of local politicians to question the CDC and the ADA. The supporters of fluoridation usually have little or no interest in engaging in public debate. Instead, the strategy is to ignore or ridicule anyone opposed to injecting the industrial pollutant fluoride into public water supplies.

Over 250 million Americans have untreated hazardous waste (fluoride) pouring from their faucets. And perhaps you and your family may be drinking. Although it is untreated hazardous waste, fluoridation promoters will tell you it is highly diluted. That's true! With your drinking water!

Rarely do I meet anyone, including dentists and physicians, who knows the truth about where the fluoride in drinking water comes from. Most people assume that it is pharmaceutical-grade – a highly refined

---

8. https://www.nytimes.com/1995/03/10/obituaries/edward-ber-
nays-father-public-relations-leader-opinion-making-dies-103.
html

and purified product. When I explain the source, their usual first response is, "Well, yes, the fluoride may come from hazardous waste, but it's treated, refined, or purified before it's added to the water supply, right?"

People want to believe this because thinking otherwise would be very disturbing. But the truth is as I previously described it. The fluoride-rich hazardous waste is not treated. It is not refined. It is not purified.

Why should any drug be added to public drinking water supplies in a country founded on individual rights and freedom to choose? Fluoride is the only chemical added to public water supplies intended to treat the people drinking it and not the water itself!

In places where fluoridation has been prevented or has ended, there have been enough well-informed people to do something about it. Those of us who oppose water fluoridation hope that many more people will begin to care about these suppressed and hidden facts concerning fluoridation.

If you are concerned about this, I recommend you read *The Case Against Fluoride* and go to the website fluoridealert.org, which is the home base for the Fluoride Action Network. I hope you are ready to get involved in making this long-overdue change in your community.

CHAPTER 13

Oral Hygiene that Promotes a Healthy Terrain

Oil pulling is a self-care practice that has been around for centuries. Ayurvedic medicine (from India) teaches that oil pulling improves oral and systemic health (your terrain). This practice involves using about a tablespoon of good-quality oil, such as castor, sesame, or sunflower (my preference is castor oil), as you would a mouthwash. I recommend oil pulling for "pulling" infection and toxicity out of the teeth, gums, and other tissues in the mouth.

My clinical experience has taught me that oil pulling is especially valuable for

✓ Treating gum infections and inflammation

✓ Preventing or reducing plaque dental plaque

✓ Providing a soothing and healing effect on all soft tissues of the mouth

✓ Preventing or reducing bad breath

As a holistic practitioner I know that improving oral health will also improve overall health. If you already have a dentally clean mouth (NO shiny metals, root canals, tooth decay, gum disease, or other stress factors), oil pulling can provide valuable health protection for your mouth and body.

Even if you have a dentally dirty mouth (sources of infection and toxicity), oil pulling can have protective and even therapeutic value for you. The more dental problems someone has, the more value oil pulling can provide as it helps reduce toxicity in the mouth and throughout the body.

How to Use Oil Pulling to Improve Your Health

Castor, sesame, and sunflower oils are traditionally recommended for oil pulling. Other oils, such as coconut and olive oil, can be used as substitutes for short periods, but I think it's best to stick with the traditional oils for best results.

Once you have your oil...

1. Put about one tablespoon of oil in your mouth and gently swish the oil around in your mouth. DO NOT SWALLOW THE OIL! If you can do oil pulling without difficulty, continue for at least 10 minutes, but 15 to 20 minutes is traditionally considered optimum. If the procedure makes you gag and you can't do it for 10 minutes, do it for as long as possible. Even doing it for a minute can have some value, and

if you practice doing it daily, or at least every other day, you should be able to work up to the recommended 10 to 20 minutes.

2. SPIT OUT THE OIL AS THOROUGHLY AS YOU CAN after swishing as long as you can tolerate without exceeding 20 minutes.

3. Thoroughly rinse your mouth with water, spit that out, and you are done. (Rinsing with warm water works best; you may want to do it several times so your mouth feels thoroughly rinsed.) I recommend spitting the oil directly into a trash container to avoid clogging your bathroom or kitchen sink drain. If you spit it out in a sink, rinse it with hot water and a squirt of liquid soap.

Now that you understand the basic procedure, here are some other suggestions I want to share. I recommend using the best-quality oil; ideally, an organic castor or sesame oil pressed from raw, untoasted seeds. It is best to use an oil that comes in a dark glass bottle because oils in general – and these oils in particular – can be damaged to some degree by exposure to light. Always refrigerate the oil after opening the bottle, regardless of whether the label advises doing so.

It is best to do oil pulling on an empty stomach (before eating or drinking anything other than water) because if it is done too soon after consuming digestible food, it can produce a feeling of nausea.

The oral hygiene protocol I recommend to my patients (and follow myself) is a four-step process:

1. Brush your teeth

2. "Polish," or wipe, all the surfaces of your teeth with a clean gauze, thin towel, or a piece of cloth

3. Foss

4. Finish with oil-pulling

If you have a dentally clean mouth, doing oil pulling for 10 minutes once a day or even every other day should be enough.

If you have a dentally dirty mouth, I recommend oil pulling at least once daily, but twice daily (morning and night) is better. Also, it would be ideal to do two rounds of oil pulling back to back – the first round shorter and the second round longer. Specifically, do an initial five-minute round, thoroughly spit out the oil, and rinse your mouth. Next, take a fresh oil dose and do your second round for 10 to 20 minutes.

Doing a round of oil pulling for at most 20 minutes can be counterproductive. Remember that the oil has a cleansing effect on your mouth, and what your mouth is being cleansed of is being transferred into the oil, so don't leave it in your mouth too long.

Feel free to take care of some other things while doing oil pulling, but always be attentive to NOT SWALLOWING THE OIL!

I have one last suggestion I want to share with you. It involves using oil pulling and a sauna as part of a more comprehensive approach to better health. A sauna induces sweating in a way that can be highly effective in helping the body to excrete toxic metals and chemicals through the skin.

An Even More Powerful Protocol

Here is the specific protocol that I have personally benefited from:

1. I spend 10 to 15 minutes in a sauna.

2. Then I get out of the sauna and shower to thoroughly rinse off my sweat and its toxins.

3. While still wet from my shower, I go back to the sauna, but before I get in, I take a mouthful of oil to do oil pulling while in the sauna.

4. I get another 10 to 15 minutes of sauna-induced sweating that is now complemented by oil pulling.

5. I leave the sauna, thoroughly spit out the oil, rinse my mouth, and then finish with another shower.

6. I then drink some glass-bottled spring water and fresh organic (primarily green) vegetable juice to replace the water and electrolyte minerals I sweated out. The juice is delicious and refreshing, and I appreciate the cleansing effect of green-vegetable nutrition.

CHAPTER 14

Ozone Therapy: A Powerful, Natural Infection Fighter

Ozone is a form of oxygen that is often associated with air pollution. The reality is that ozone is a natural air purifier because it can transform harmful pollutants in the air into compounds that are much better for health and the environment. Ozone also has natural anti-microbial properties that make it a perfect substance for clearing up infections in the body, especially in the mouth.

The oxygen molecule we breathe comprises two oxygen atoms bonded by electrons they share. For this reason, the chemical notation for this oxygen is O_2. Ozone is also made up of oxygen atoms. Rather than two atoms, however, ozone has three. Its chemical notation is O_3.

Ozone is formed in the stratosphere when oxygen molecules are exposed to solar radiation, causing the two oxygen atoms in the oxygen molecule to separate.

When a free oxygen atom joins with another oxygen molecule, it forms ozone. A layer of this gas in the earth's outer atmosphere protects the planet from the sun's harmful rays.

When nitrogen oxides interact with volatile organic compounds in sunlight, ozone can be created at the earth's surface. Due to temperature inversions, ozone formed in this way can accumulate in smog and irritate the lungs and eyes. Although ozone does not cause pollution, it is easy to measure accurately and is therefore used and quoted as an indicator of environmental pollution.

Ozone was first synthesized in the mid 1800s. The first uses were technological, the most common being water purification. As a powerful oxidant, ozone can destroy pathogens with little or no antioxidant enzymes in their cell membranes, such as bacteria, fungi, viruses, and parasites. Without this antioxidant protection, ozone quickly degrades the pathogen's cell membrane, causing it to rupture and die. Healthy cells have antioxidant enzymes in their cell membranes and are not harmed by therapeutic ozone levels.

The Medical Uses of Ozone

Ozone has been used to treat cancer, autoimmune diseases, chronic infections, allergies, sinusitis, intestinal disorders, ear infections, dental problems, arthritis, chronic pain, and degenerative backs.

Medical ozone is generated by passing pure oxygen through an electric energy field in a "corona discharge generator." This energy splits some of the oxygen molecules, and what emerges from the other side is a mixture of oxygen and ozone. Ozone comprises only two to five percent of the gas discharged by the generator. The rest is oxygen. Because ozone is somewhat unstable, it quickly breaks down at room temperature. About half of the ozone present returns to oxygen every hour at room temperature (called the half-life). So after an hour, only about half the ozone remains; in two hours, about one quarter, etc. Cooling the ozone slows this process of decay.

The ozone/oxygen gas is infused into water (ozonated) for patient care. This allows the dentist to treat all oral infections. It is the perfect irrigation solution for periodontics (issues relating to the gums) and endodontics (issues relating to the dental pulp). For operative dentistry, ozone gas is used to treat areas such as carious dentin, dentinal tubules, accessory canals, and periodontal pockets where no other antibiotic or disinfectant can reach.

Ozonated water is used in hygienic applications to protect patients and staff, as well as a pretreatment rinse for patients. It is also used in water-supply bottles and ultrasonic water reservoirs. This natural disinfectant is a practical, non-invasive treatment for periodontal disease since it can reach below the gum line to destroy bacteria.

Ozonated gas is used before placing dental restorations (fillings, inlays, onlays or crowns) because it enhances bonding strength, decreases post-operative sensitivity.

Ozone is administered through various methods, including autohemotherapy (reintroduction of ozone-infused blood), injection of gas, insufflation with gas (rectal, vaginal, auricular), irrigation with ozonated water, inhalation, and topically with ozonated oil. Because of its remarkable antiseptic qualities, ozone was used successfully to treat infected wounds during the First World War. It was first used medically extensively in Germany in the early 1950s. Today, ozone therapy is standard throughout Europe and has gradually spread to the United States over the last 25 years. It continues to be a part of the medical mainstream in Germany, Russia, and Cuba. And more than 40 international organizations represent around 30,000 physicians who use ozone in their daily practice.

A German dentist first used dental ozone therapy in Zurich, Switzerland, many years ago. However, in this country, ozone therapy is primarily used in holistic dentistry. The results have been excellent. It can be used clinically for restorative periodontal, endodontic, surgical, and dental hygiene procedures. It treats mild and acute infections (canker sores, periodontal disease, cavities, tooth decay, etc.).

Is Medical Ozone Use Safe?

Ozone can be toxic to living organisms at excessive concentrations. However, this is true of most substances given in quantities higher than the body can tolerate. Medical treatment with ozone is entirely safe when it involves very specific and controlled dosage levels and proper administration methods.

Simply smelling ozone (ozone is responsible for the fresh smell after a thunderstorm) does not pose a health threat, especially the small amount of ozone released as hoses are changed, syringes are purged, or water is being ozonated. In addition, as ozonated water does its disinfectant work, it decomposes into the harmless elements of water and oxygen. There are no drug residues and no side effects.

There are hundreds of published research studies on the use of ozone in dental procedures. The book *Ozone: The Revolution in Dentistry*, edited by Edward Lynch, has 132 studies on using ozone for various dental problems. Ozone is a powerful oxidant, so those who use it must employ safe practices, but when used properly, it is safe and effective. Ozone overexposure to dental patients can be easily mitigated by nasal oxygen administration.

Three Case Studies

It is no wonder that dentists are using this powerful tool in their offices. Here are three case studies from my practice that illustrate how effective ozone therapy can be:

Patient #1

This patient called for an emergency appointment due to much pain and bleeding under her bridge. The patient was experiencing acute symptoms and was concerned she might lose the teeth holding the bridge in place. After clinical examination and X-rays, the treatment of choice was ozone therapy. Following the ozone therapy, the pain immediately subsided, and the patient was sent home.

Patient #2

A woman experiencing TMJ pain (temporomandibular disorder in her jaw) bit her cheek and had an infection with swollen lymph nodes and severe pain. After the first treatment with ozone therapy, the patient could sleep through the night for the first time in a week. After the second treatment, she could eat and chew without discomfort. After the third treatment, the sore on her cheek healed, and the problem was resolved.

Patient #3

A patient had a lesion on her tongue that she was advised to have biopsied. After refusing a biopsy, the patient came to our office for help. After three ozone therapy treatments, the lesion was resolved, and the patient did not need a biopsy or further assistance.

In Summary

As these cases indicate, ozone therapy eases pain, reduces infection, prepares tooth surfaces, and so much more. It has promising applications and many dentists are using it now with remarkable results.

CHAPTER 15

Laser Dentistry: A Better Way

LASER is an acronym for Light Amplification by the Stimulated Emission of Radiation. It is a way of focusing light and harnessing the energy that it contains for many purposes. The first laser was constructed by Dr. Theodore Maiman, a physicist at Hughes Electric Corporation in California, in 1960.

Lasers were first used in dentistry in 1964 to remove hard tissue (called ablationablation), such as the infected portion of a tooth or bone. Although there were several advantages over drilling, early lasers were not ideal because the heat they generated tended to cause cracks and carbonization in the dental pulp.

Since the first dental applications, laser technology has improved tremendously. Current lasers provide much better temperature and depth of penetration cont rol and allows superior treatment of both hard (tooth/bone) and soft tissue. For periodontal procedures, these lasers provide higher power for faster cutting speed, improved hemostasis (cessation of bleeding), quick ablation, and reduced pain. When used as a single treatment or for complementing surgical procedures, these lasers remove soft tissue, hard tissue, and biofilms without causing thermal damage to adjacent tissues. They also diminish the need for local anesthesia, minimize post-operative pain, and decrease recovery time.

In surgical procedures, good hemostasis, ideal bone healing, are achieved when lasers are used. Other benefits include selective and exact interaction with tissues-which results in less trauma, the ability to lower the bacterial load in the surgical field, reduced inflammation, and stimulation of new fibroblasts and osteoblasts for improved healing. Lasers have also been instrumental in managing gingival tissues and for periodontal pocket therapy, osseous surgery, and implant therapy.

Compared to a scalpel, lasers produce excellent coagulation, reduce pathogens, temporarily seal nerve endings and lymphatic vessels, and potentially eliminate the need for sutures with less scar formation.

When used for hard-tissue applications, lasers eliminate vibrations, the sound of dental drills, and microfractures and alleviate the stress that patients associate with high-speed handpieces. Restoratively speaking, and compared to a dentist's drill, lasers produce no smear layer on dentin or bone, no micro-fracturing of enamel, and simultaneously disinfect hard-tissue surfaces.

Diagnostic applications include detecting carious lesions and calculus, temporarily increasing local blood circulation, and temporarily relieving minor aches and pains.

The field of laser-based photochemical reactions holds great promise for additional applications, particularly for targeting specific cells, pathogens, or molecules. Specific laser technologies will become even more essential components of contemporary dental practice.

Summary of Dental Laser Advantages

1. **Minimally invasive.** Laser "drilling" provides a precise and gentle way to remove only the decayed portions of a tooth, infected bone, and soft tissues. Laser "drilling" produces much less discomfort, meaning less anesthetic need.

2. **Promotes faster healing**: Because of its speed and precision, laser surgeries on soft tissue preserve more healthy tissue, produce less bleeding, and require fewer sutures. Extractions are less traumatic when performed with a laser; there is less bone loss and quicker wound healing, leading to faster and more predictable implants. In addition, the light and heat generated by the laser have powerful disinfectant properties that reduce the chance of infection and speed recovery.

3. **No traditional drilling sounds or vibration.** Lasers operate without the shrill noise of a conventional drill and do not cause any vibration, so tooth preparation is faster, quieter, and much less stress-producing.

4. **Shorter treatment time.** Usually, dental procedures performed with lasers take less time than those using traditional dental tools. This means

less trauma for the patient and quicker recovery times.

5. **Reduction of tooth sensitivity.** Conventionally-treated teeth can produce short, sharp pain when exposed dentin (the portion of the tooth under the enamel) comes in contact with heat, cold, touch, or certain foods. This sensitivity can be greatly minimized when teeth are treated with lasers. The properties of the light can recrystallize the dentin, which produces a nonporous surface that seals off the dentinal tubules that transmit the pain signals and provide additional protection to the treated tooth.

CHAPTER 16

Hyperbaric Therapy: A Game Changer

Some of the most fundamental therapeutics in my practice utilize oxygen gas. I keep oxygen on hand for medical emergencies and use ozone as a disinfectant and antiseptic. Because my instinct (based upon my intuition and reinforced by my experience) favors treatment involving oxygen in one form or another, I often (almost daily) suggest Hyperbaric Oxygen Therapy (HBOT) to patients when appropriate.

Traditional HBOT administers pure, pressurized oxygen as an adjunctive therapy to decrease inflammation in chronic burn wounds. Generally, HBOT is delivered in a monoplace (type A) chamber or a multiplace (type B) chamber with an atmosphere of 100% oxygen under pressures from 1.5 to 3 atmosphere absolute (ATA) for a limited time in a series of treatment sessions. In a monoplace chamber, one patient is enveloped in an atmosphere of pure, compressed oxygen. In a multiplace chamber, multiple patients are exposed to a normal

(78% nitrogen and 21% oxygen) but pressurized atmo-sphere while each patient breathes pressurized 100% oxygen through a face mask or hood.

High-pressure gas therapy was initially used to treat deep sea diver decompression injuries (the bends) caused by divers ascending too quickly. However, the mechanisms that make HBOT an effective treatment for decompression sickness (arterial gas embolism) are different from the mechanisms that make HBOT an effective treatment for the following chronic wounds and infections:

✓ Carbon monoxide poisoning (when enough carbon monoxide builds up in the blood and leads to severe tissue damage or death)

✓ Concussion (type of traumatic brain injury caused by a bump, blow, or jolt to the head or by a hit to the body)

✓ Delayed radiation injury (most commonly occurs in tumor treatment sites in the head, neck, breast, chest, and pelvis)

✓ Diabetic ulcers (an open sore or wound that occurs in diabetes patients)

✓ Gangrene (dead tissue caused by an infection or lack of blood flow)

✓ Infective endocarditis (infection caused by bacteria that enter the bloodstream and settle in the heart lining, a heart valve, or a blood vessel)

✓ Lyme disease (tick-borne illness caused by the bacterium Borrelia burgdorferi)

✓ Necrotizing fasciitis (a severe bacterial infection that destroys the tissue under the skin)

✓ Osteomyelitis (bone infection)

✓ Osteonecrosis (death of bone tissue due to a lack of blood supply)

✓ Periodontitis (significant bone loss around teeth)

Additionally, HBOT is an effective treatment for many more conditions related to the heart, brain (stroke), cancer, and other neurological and auto-immune disorders.

Although most hospitals are equipped with hyperbaric chambers, these devices are rarely used beyond treating burn injuries because HBOT is not typically included in the standards of care for many other conditions where HBOT is highly effective. As a result, doctors are reluctant to employ HBOT more widely, and insurance companies rarely cover the cost of HBOT beyond use as a treatment or last resort for chronic burns or infections.

Most hospitals have a hyperbaric chamber (usually in the burn unit) as a standby resource of last resort – when drugs or antibiotics fail to achieve the desired results. This is upside-down to my way of thinking. Although counterintuitive to me, traditional dental treatment protocols usually begin with drugs, and rarely, if ever, is HBOT suggested for oral or dental infections. Those interested in pursuing HBOT will have an uphill battle, especially patients needing insurance coverage for immediate HBOT.

Thank goodness physicians and hospitals are available for initial diagnosis and emergencies. But once a crisis has passed or a diagnosis has been made, you must assert yourself and take responsibility for your treatment to achieve the best possible outcome. As a dentist with years of practice helping people, I know firsthand that a mouth free of toxic material and infection yet full of healthy micro-organisms is a prerequisite for gut and overall health. And HBOT, unlike medication, is compatible with maintaining a healthy oral terrain. Your gut is your second brain, and utilizing food as your medicine ensures optimal gut terrain. A clean mouth and gut with beneficial flora are vital to your well-being.

NOTE: *As a physician and a patient, I have found a monoplace (type A, in particular, Sechrist Industries brand) chamber to be most effective for dental needs using 100% oxygen under pressures from 1.5 to 2 atmospheres (ATA) for at least an hour for a minimum series of ten treatment sessions. If treatment in a monoplace chamber is unavailable, a multiplace (type B) chamber will suffice. When entering a monoplace chamber, be sure to remove all jewelry, wear only cotton clothing, and never bring other objects of any kind into the chamber. A pure oxygen atmosphere makes many commonplace materials highly flammable, and one must carefully adhere to strict protocols designed to assure your safety in a 100% oxygen environment.*Regarding what I know is a fundamentally important understanding of human metabolism and nutrition, I would also like to express our appreciation for the contributions made by Dr. George Watson, Dr. William Donald Kelley, Dr. Rudolf Wiley and, especially, William Wolcott. I also appreciate the work of Dr. Nicholas Gonzalez, Dr. Harold Kristal and Dodie Anderson.

CHAPTER 17

3-Way Care: How Practitioners Should Cooperate

A Note to Readers

Although I have been a holistic dentist for many years, my practice has been enriched by working with Dr. Joseph Grasso, an osteopathic physician, and Jim Marlowe, whose advice on nutrition has been invaluable to both of us.

By now, those of you who have read the earlier chapters of my book know I believe in an integrative approach to health. That means treating the body as a whole and realizing that what happens in your mouth may have effects elsewhere, and what happens in other parts of your body may affect your mouth.

So, in addition to asking several of my patients to comment on what's different about seeing a holistic dentist, I joined with Dr. Grasso in a discussion about a few cases in which we have referred patients to each other, as well as questions about how a discovery in one part of the body can lead to better health in another area.

I hope you enjoy the interview.

— Dr. Lina Garcia

Interviewer: Dr. Garcia, although you have different practices, each of you is concerned with the total health of your patients, so let's start on that note. In treating teeth and gum issues and looking at the relationship between dental problems and ill-health manifestations elsewhere in the body, what leads you to refer patients to an osteopathic physician?

Dr. Garcia: One of the first things I do is a medical history. I note what drugs my patients may be taking (pharmaceutical or recreational) and their history of surgery, trauma, and related concerns. If patients have compromised immune system, for example, they're more prone to root-canal problems or periodontal (gum) disease.

It's almost like working as a detective. A pain in the jaw may indicate inflammation elsewhere in the body. Dr. Grasso can help patients discontinue harmful drugs and adopt a healthier lifestyle, including exercise. A change in diet also may be crucial, and nutrition advice needed from Jim Marlowe.

Interviewer: Dr. Grasso, as an osteopathic physician who treats the whole patient – including the nervous, circulatory, and endocrine systems and psyche – what kinds of things would lead you to refer patients to a holistic dentist?

Dr. Grasso: Most medical and even alternative physicians don't consider asking about their patient's dental history, but in my office, a dental history, along with all other medical issues, is a routine part of what we ask new patients. I must consider all possibilities contributing to a patient's problem. That includes dental issues, such as root canals, periodontal disease, implants, mercury-amalgam fillings, and orthodontics.

Interviewer: Dr. Garcia, are there any special diagnostic tests or practices you use that conventional dentists don't use?

Dr. Garcia: Besides the usual tests that conventional dentists rely on, I use a live microscopy slide to determine whether a patient's immune system is healthy. A little plaque is taken from the patient's mouth and put under a microscope to look for beneficial or pathogenic bacteria, parasites, viruses, or yeast.

I also use homeopathic remedies, laser, hyperbaric therapy, and I use ozone therapy to kill pathogens in a patient's mouth.

I use ozone therapy to kill pathogens in a patient's mouth. I use Hyperbaric Oxygen treatment to promote long-term healing. And I also use laser technology to improve dental procedure outcomes.

Interviewer: Dr. Grasso, what distinguishes your treatment approach from conventional doctors?

Dr. Grasso: In my practice, looking at the whole patient, not just the disease, is essential. I look at a patient from a place of health; despite an illness, there is always something healthy I can tap into to facilitate healing.

As osteopathic physicians, we use our hands and perceptual abilities, which take years to develop, as instruments to open doorways that facilitate healing. It is much more than manipulating different parts of the body or doing therapy on the musculoskeletal system. We can access all body systems, including the nervous, circulatory, respiratory, endocrine, reproductive, musculoskeletal, and immune systems. We work with normal functions in the body to facilitate healing.

Interviewer: Dr. Garcia, would you walk through a couple of cases in which you referred a patient to Dr. Grasso and Jim Marlowe?

Dr. Garcia: Certainly. One of my patients was a 50-year-old man with infected teeth, gum disease, and heart problems. He also had high blood pressure, and I was concerned that his dental problems were related to his blood pressure and heart conditions. So, I referred him to Dr. Grasso and suggested he also get nutritional advice from Jim Marlowe.

Dr. Grasso treated the patient's blood pressure and cholesterol problems while eliminating the need for medications related to those problems. This patient was also sensitive to gluten and was advised to eliminate sugar and gluten from his diet. He added vegetable juice to his daily intake regimen, changed his eating habits, and improved his health dramatically.

Another case was a 38-year-old woman with root canals and mercury-amalgam fillings. She was also diagnosed with rheumatoid arthritis, generalized joint pain in her hands and knees, and TMJ pain (involving jaw movement).

After removing her root canals and mercury fillings, I referred her to Dr. Grasso because she needed osteopathic treatment to relieve her pain and overcome her dependence on drugs.

This patient also received nutritional advice from Jim Marlowe, eliminated sugar from her diet, and added vegetable juice, fish, and poultry.

Her symptoms subsided with the combination of dental care, osteopathic help, and nutritional advice, and she is now living a normal life.

Interviewer: Dr. Grasso, I'd like to ask you the same question. Would you relate a couple of times when you referred a patient to Dr. Garcia and Jim Marlowe?

Dr. Grasso: I treated a middle-aged woman with severe post-menopausal symptoms, migraine headaches, and chronic pain in her lower back, hip, and neck. As an osteopath, it's my job to examine all aspects of a patient. In doing so, I learned about her injury problems and some emotional baggage she had been carrying for years.

In addition, she had a mouth full of metals and mercury fillings that further aggravated her condition. The toxins in her mouth compromised her weakened immune system and contributed to inflammation in various parts of her body.

I referred her to Dr. Garcia, who cleaned up her mouth and replaced everything with biocompatible materials. When she returned to my office, there was a significant increase in her vitality and a dramatic improvement in her immune system. I then successfully addressed some of her other problems, and her migraines have greatly diminished, while her chronic pain has been reduced.

Her menopausal symptoms are also improving, and she has followed a sound, inflammation-free nutrition program that contributed to our success.

Another one of my patients was a 72-year-old woman who complained of dizziness and heart palpitations. Along with these symptoms, which she thought began after a root canal, she had experienced pain in her neck and numbness in her legs for several years.

The patient first went to see Dr. Garcia because her primary care physician denied there was a relationship between her recent problems and the root canal procedure. After evaluating this patient, Dr. Garcia referred her to my office for osteopathic treatment.

While easing this patient's neck and leg problems, I weaned her off a medication to control the palpitations since tests indicated her heart was working normally. I also referred her for a nutritional evaluation, and her condition gradually improved enough to allow Dr. Garcia to extract the root-canal tooth. Following the extraction, the patient significantly reduced her dizziness and palpitations.

In this case, the interesting dynamic is that Dr. Garcia and I worked very closely to improve this patient's health. The osteopathic treatment and nutritional support got her to a place where she was ready to have the root-canal tooth extracted.

Interviewer: Dr. Garcia, are there new developments or treatments on the horizon that may help holistic dentists treat patients in the future?

Dr. Garcia: I hope to see increasing use of microscopy slides in which plaque is taken from a patient's mouth and examined under a microscope to determine the health of a patient's immune system.

I also hope to see a wider use of ozone therapy in which a machine converts oxygen in a tank to ozone and infuses it into a patient's mouth to kill pathogens. And finally, I hope to see more frequent use of homeopathic remedies, supplements and using food as medicine instead of drugs.

Another technology that is seeing tremendous growth and acceptance is using lasers to quickly, quietly, and virtually painlessly remove dental caries (cavities). Now, lasers have been refined to where surgery can be performed rapidly and with much less trauma, pain, and recovery time. I believe the less trauma inflicted on teeth and gums, the better the patient outcome.

I also hope to see an increase in the use of Hyperbaric Oxygen Therapy (HBOT) in cases where additional effort is required for long-term healing.

Interviewer: Dr. Grasso, how about in the osteopathic realm? Are there new developments or treatments on the horizon that may help physicians treat patients in the future?

Dr. Grasso: I hope that all healthcare practitioners learn to be better listeners and spend more time observing the whole patient and not just their symptoms or disease. This includes taking a complete medical history, including an in-depth dental history.

In addition, I would love to see all medical schools demand intensive study of nutrition. Hippocrates, the father of modern medicine, said, "Let food be thy medicine." As a culture, we are severely diminished in this regard and need to realize, as we have in our (osteopathic) practices, that most health conditions can be relieved, cured, or prevented with proper nutrition.

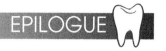

A Powerful Confirmation of a Vital Reality

Even while writing about the intimate relationship between the health of one's mouth and the health of one's body, this reality was brought home to me in a painful, somewhat humbling way. As I was working through the final edits of *Cleaner Mouth, Longer Life*, I developed acute, persistent pain in my left hand near my thumb.

Generally, this type of pain resolves quickly because my nutrition and self-care habits are conducive to self-healing. In this case, the pain wouldn't go away, causing me great difficulty opening containers and lifting heavy objects. Doing anything that required using my left thumb was uncomfortable, and dental work that required wearing tight-fitting gloves became much more painful – almost debilitating.

The pain wouldn't go away, and after about five months, the gum on the palate of my upper left wisdom tooth began to hurt, too. At this point, I began to get suspicious. I constantly teach my patients to look for chronic aches and pains attributable to oral problems, and now I needed to teach myself. I was confused, however, since that wisdom tooth showed no signs of external damage. Nevertheless, as my left-hand pain increased, so did the pain around my wisdom tooth as I brushed and polished my teeth every night.

Although it is easier for me to be more attentive to the needs of my patients than my own, about three months after the onset of the wisdom tooth pain, I decided something more than a visual examination of my wisdom tooth (which revealed no signs of external damage or decay) was in order. An X-ray revealed that my wisdom tooth had **internal resorption** (a type of disintegration of the tooth from within that eventually destroys the surrounding tooth structure).

The tooth needed to come out because it was dying. Within a few hours of the extraction, the pain in my thumb started to fade away. After about a week, the left hand pain completely disappeared. I could open containers, lift heavy items, and work in tight-fitting gloves since my thumb had ultimately returned to normal.

Of course, the pain resolved; that's what I teach. I have observed that in patients for 40 years, and that's one of the main points of this book. For decades, I have witnessed the connection between teeth and the rest of the body, but now this living connection has been vali-dated in my own experience – even as I was finishing this book.

Every time something strange happens within the body, it is essential to correlate that to the oral cavity condition – teeth, gums, jawbone – and the sinuses. Ensuring our nutrition, mental, and spiritual habits support our healing is essential.

If there is an oral issue, the rest of the body is most likely being challenged, and vice versa. My recent experience with wisdom-tooth internal reabsorption further assures that everything written in this book is precise, clear, and worthy of serious consideration when diagnosing any health issue.

If this book has been helpful to you, consider getting my second book, *Holistic Inquiry*. People concerned about their health and their loved ones must learn to be proactive health advocates in a system more concerned for its protection and profits than for the patients it is supposed to serve. My years of work in the healthcare system, as well as my experience with life-threatening Reversible Cerebral Vasoconstriction Syndrome (RCVS) and subarachnoid hemorrhage, taught me the necessity of being able to ask the right questions of medical professionals in the navigation of the current healthcare system. *Holistic Inquiry* has been written to help you do just that.

The human body is an amazing organism designed for self-healing. May you discover and employ ways to enable you to cooperate with it as you move toward better health and wellness.

-- Lina Garcia

The Food Diary

General Instructions

Keeping a food diary for as little as one week can provide unique insights into your optimum metabolic balance. It will also help you identify foods that your body is sensitive to, does not process well, or genuinely produces positive benefits.

As you begin to list the foods you eat at each meal and how your body responds to each meal, you will become more attuned to how your body functions. Over a few days, you will begin to see patterns that will help you weed out those foods that hinder your moods, energy, and mental clarity and those that improve them.

One of the primary goals of keeping this diary is to bring you to the point where evaluating your body's response to various foods and eating styles becomes automatic. At that point, you are "listening to your body."

If you have mixed results, ensure you have read Chapter 10, or if you have already read it, you should reread it.

The diary is also recommended if you follow one of the Metabolic Tendency Plans (see Chapter 11) to evaluate and adjust your carbohydrate-to-protein/fat ratio.

As mentioned in Chapter 11, you can expect to see the following benefits from eating in harmony with your metabolic tendencies, and by eliminating those foods your body has difficulty processing:

- ✓ More energy with the consumption of less food
- ✓ More alertness, improved mental clarity, better mood
- ✓ Improved immunity
- ✓ Less tendency to overeat and movement toward your ideal weight
- ✓ Better response to exercise
- ✓ Healthier teeth and gums

Note: although the Daily Food Diary on the page at right is covered by our copyright, you have permission to use and copy it as needed for personal use only.

Specific Instructions

Before you eat each meal, complete the assessment by rating the mood, energy, mental clarity, and satisfaction level you may be experiencing at that time. This will provide the necessary feedback for how your body responded to those foods you ate at your last meal.

You will also notice physical factors, such as physical strength, stuffy or clear sinuses, constipation, particular muscle/joint aches, headaches, lightheadedness, relief of pain, vision clarity, etc. It would be best if

Listening to Your Body
Daily Food Diary

Date

BREAKFAST

BEFORE-Breakfast Assessment *(Circle rating - Excellent=5 to Terrible=0):*

Mood.. 5   4   3   2   1   0

Energy 5   4   3   2   1   0

Mental Clarity.......................... 5   4   3   2   1   0

Time_____ What did you eat for BREAKFAST

LUNCH

BEFORE-Lunch Breakfast Assessment ..... *(Circle rating):*

Mood 5   4   3   2   1   0

Energy...................................... 5   4   3   2   1   0

Mental Clarity............................ 5   4   3   2   1   0

Satisfaction Level w/ Breakfast   5 · 4   3   2   1   0

List any cravings you experienced after Breakfast:

Time_____ What did you eat for LUNCH?

DINNER

BEFORE-Dinner Lunch Assessment .... *(Circle rating):*

Mood 5   4   3   2   1   0

Energy...................................... 5   4   3   2   1   0

Mental Clarity............................ 5   4   3   2   1   0

Satisfaction Level w/ Lunch...... 5   4   3   2   1   0

List any cravings you experienced after Breakfast:

Time_____ What did you eat for DINNER?

BEDTIME

BEFORE-Bedtime Dinner Assessment .... *(Circle rating):*

Mood 5   4   3   2   1   0

Energy...................................... 5   4   3   2   1   0

Mental Clarity............................ 5   4   3   2   1   0

Satisfaction Level w/ Dinner..... 5   4   3   2   1   0

Overall satisfaction with today 5   4   3   2   1   0

Comments or observations for the day

you also tracked these, but the rated factors will give you a quick way to see general patterns.

Anytime you see ratings below a three, consider eliminating one or more of the foods you ate at the previous meal. Ultimately, you want to eat the foods that keep you in a four or five-rating zone. At that point, you will begin to experience many of the benefits listed above.

I hope you will soon know that "food is your best medicine."

Questions to Help Identify a Holistic Dentist

Finding a genuinely holistic dentist can be challenging. Many dentists consider themselves holistic simply because they replace amalgam fillings or refuse to perform root canals. Indeed, these are part of the profile, but there is much more. The ultimate question is whether they consider the entire being, including nutrition, general health, medical history, dental history, and stress levels, among other things, before deciding how to treat the patient.

Although no two dentists practice their profession the same way, here is a list of questions you should ask prospective dentists to help you decide whether they can help you with your particular dental and general health needs.

Remember, however, these questions should be asked in a non-adversarial way. The idea is to get potential dentists to provide their genuine opinions. Then, when you understand where they are coming from, you can make an informed decision. This process will work best when the one you are interviewing does not know your opinion.

Q: How much do you think my general health is related to my dental health?

Comment: If you don't get a clear answer, you are not talking to a holistic practitioner.

Q: Some say silver filling can cause health problems over time. Do you think that is true?

Comment: If the dentist says "yes," Here is a follow-up question:

Q: Do you recommend the removal of silver fillings, and if so, how do you do that?

Comment: If a dentist does not use extreme measures to reduce exposure to mercury vapor during removal, he or she does not fully understand the danger, and this is not someone you want to do this kind of work.

Q: I've heard that some dentists don't think there should be any metal fillings, crowns, bridgework, or implants in the mouth. Do you think that is true?

Comment: It is important to avoid having metal dental work in the mouth. However, if you just need routine dental work, this wouldn't necessarily disqualify a dentist.

Q: How much dental and medical history do you get from a new patient before doing work?

Comment: If the answer is little or none, this dentist is not concerned with the whole person.

Q: Do you routinely refer patients to an osteopath, medical doctor, or nutritionist for conditions that may be related to a patient's dental problems?

Comment: If you don't get a solid "yes" to this question, you are not talking to a holistic practitioner.

Q: Do you perform root canals or refer them to an endodontist?

Comment: If the dentist does either, you consider another provider.

Q: Do you routinely use ceramic inlays or onlays to fill cavities?

Comment: If the dentist does not use inlays or onlays to treat cavities, he or she is most likely using composite fillings. These plastic fillings leach potentially harmful chemicals into the body, and because they are not exceptionally durable, they often crack or break and require replacement in the future.

Reading Resources by Chapter

- Chapter 4 -
How Should You Care for Cavities and Chipped Teeth

Clifford, Walter J. Personal Communications, June 13, 2012.

Clifford, Walter J. Personal Communications, Sept. 29, 2009.

Chaturvedi, T.P. An Overview of the Corrosion Aspect of Dental Implants (Titanium And Its Alloys). *Indian Journal of Dental Research*, 20(1), 2009. Pp 91-98.

Depprich, R.; Zipprich, H.; Ommerborn, M.; Naujoks, C.; Wiesmann, H.P.; Kiattavorncharoen, S.; Lauer, H.C.; Meyer, U.; Kubler, N.R.; and Handschel J. Osseointegration of Zirconia Implants Compared With Titanium: An In Vivo Study. *Head & Face Medicine* 2008, 4:30.

Dorner, T.; Haas, J.; Loddenkemper, C.; von Baehr, V.; and Salama, A. Implant-Related Inflammatory Arthritis. Nature Clinical Practice *Rheumatology*, January 2006, Vol. 2, No. 1, pp. 53-56.

Hentges, Steven G. Bisphenol-A in Dental Composites. Original article at http://www.bisphenol-a.org/human/dental.html. Reproduced in 2007 by IAOMT at www.iaomt.org. Last accessed Sept. 8, 2009.

Hyams B.L. and Ballon H.C. *Dissimilar Metals in the Mouth as a Possible Cause of Otherwise Unexplainable Symptoms.* Can. M. J. 29: 488, 1932.

Ionescu, J.G.; Novotny, J; Stejskal, V.D.; Latsch, A.; Blaurock-Busch, E.; Eisenmann-Klein, M. Increased levels of Transition Metals in Breast Cancer Tissue. *Neuro Endocrinol Lett.* 2006; 27(Suppl1): 36-39.

Lambrich, M.; Iglhaut, G. Comparison of the Survival Rates for Zirconia and Titanium Implants. JDI *Journal of Dental Implantology.* Vol. 24, No. 3, 2008, pp. 182-191.

Magnusson, B.; Bergman, M.; Bergman, B.; Sörenmark, R. Nickel Allergy and Nickel-Containing Dental Alloys. *Scand J Dent Res.* 1982 Apr; 90(2): 163-7.

McGuff, H.S.; Heim-Hall, J.; Holsinger, C.F.; Jones. A.A.; O'Dell, D.S.; Hafemeister, AC. Maxillary Osteosarcoma Associated with a Dental Implant: Report of a Case and Review of the Literature Regarding Implant-Related Sarcomas. *JADA,* Vol. 139. August 2008. Pp. 1052-1059.

Muller, K; Valentine-Thon, E. Hypersensitivity to Titanium: Clinical and Laboratory Evidence. *Neuroendocrinol Lett* 2006; 27(Suppl 1):31-35.

Muris, J.; Feilzer, A.J. Microanalysis of Metals in Dental Restorations as Part of a Diagnostic Approach in Metal Allergies. *Neuro Endocrinol Lett.* 2006; 27(Suppl1): 49-52.

Ndebele, Kenneth; Tchounwou, Paul B.; and McMurray, Robert W. Effects of Xenoestrogens on T Lymphocytes: Modulation of bcl-2, p53, and Apoptosis. *Int. J. Mol. Sci.* 2003, 4, 45-61.

Oliva, J.; Oliva, X.; Oliva, J.D. *One-year Follow-Up of First Consecutive 100 Zirconia Dental Implants in Humans: A Comparison of 2 Different Rough Surfaces.*

Schriever, W.; Diamond, L.E. Electromotive Forces and Electric Currents Cause by Metallic Dental Fillings. *Journal of Dental Research,* Apr 1952; vol. 31: pp. 205-229

ScienceDaily. 04/22/2008. *Chemical in Plastic Bottles Raises Some Concern, According to New Report.* Available at www.sciencedaily.com. Last accessed Sept. 8, 2009.

Stejskal, V.D.M.; Cederbrant, K.; Lindvall, A.; Forsbeck, M. MELISA - An In-Vitro Tool for the Study of Metal Allergy. *Toxic in Vitro* Vol. 8, No. 5, pp. 991-1000, 1994. Printed in Great Britain.

Stejskal, V.D.M.; Danersund, A.; Lindvall, A.; Hudecek, R.; Nordman, V.; Yaqob, A.; Mayer, W.; Bieger, W.; and Lindh, U. Metal-Specific Lymphocytes: Biomarkers of Sensitivity in Man. *Neuro Endocrinol Lett* 1999; 20:289-298.

Stejskal, V.D.; Hudecek, R.; Stejskal, J.; Sterzl, I. Diagnosis and Treatment of Metal-Induced Side Effects. *Neuro Endocrinol Lett* 2006; 27 (Suppl 1): 7-16.

Stejskal, J.; Stejskal, V.D.M. The Role of Metals in Autoimmunity and the Link to Neuroendocrinology. *Neuro Endocrinol Lett* 1999; 20:351-364.

Sterzl, I.; Prochazkova, J.; Hrda, P.; Bartova, J.; Matucha, P.; Stejskal, V.D.M. Mercury and Nickel Allergy: Risk Factors in Fatigue and Autoimmunity. *Neuro Endocrinol Lett* 1999; 20:221-228.

Valentine-Thon, E.; Muller, K.; Guzzi, G.; Kreisel, S.; Ohnsorge, P.; and Sandkamp M. LTT-MELISA® Is Clinically Relevant for Detecting and Monitoring Metal Sensitivity. *Neuro Endocrinol Lett* 2006; 27(Suppl 1):17-24.

- Chapter 5 -
Why Are Silver Fillings so Dangerous?

American Dental Association. Aug. 25, 2009. *ADA Council on Scientific Affairs Statement on Dental Amalgam.* Revised: August 2009. http://ada. org. Last accessed Sept. 2, 2009.

American Dental Association. *Principles of Ethics and Code of Professional Conduct, With Official Advisory Opinions* Revised to January 2009. www. ada.org. Last accessed Sept. 2, 2009.

The American Heritage® Medical Dictionary Copyright © 2007, 2004.

Centers for Disease Control and Prevention. *Emergency Preparedness and Response: Case Definition: Mercury (Elemental).*http://emergency.cdc. gov/agent/mercury/mercelementalcasedef.asp. Last updated March 9, 2005. Last accessed Jan. 13, 2013.

Concorde East/West Sprl. March 2012. *The Real Cost of Dental Mercury.* Available on the United Nations Environment Programme (UNEP) website at http://www.unep.org/hazardoussubstances/Portals/9/Mercury/ Documents/INC4/Submissions%20from%20NGOs/The%20Real%20 Cost%20of%20Dental%20Mercury%20Full%20Report.pdf.Last accessed Jan. 13, 2013.

International Academy of Oral Medicine and Toxicology. 2007. SAB FDA Comment. www.iaomt.org. Last accessed Sept. 1, 2009.

Kennedy, Dr. David. Jan. 23, 2009. *Less Is More in Dentistry.* One Radio Network. oneradionetwork.com. Last accessed Jan. 7, 2013. Podcast.

Lyman, Francesca. *Are "Silver" Dental Fillings Safe?* July 11, 2001. Republished on Mercola.com. http://articles.mercola.com/sites Last accessed Jan. 20, 2009.

Miller-Keane *Encyclopedia and Dictionary of Medicine, Nursing, and Allied Health,* Seventh Edition. © 2003

Mosby's *Medical Dictionary, 8th edition.* © 2009

National Council for Occupational Safety and Health. Mercury Hazards. www. coshnetwork.org/node/37. Last accessed Sept. 9, 2009.

Podzimek, Stepan; Prochazkova, Jarmila; Bultasova, Lenka; Bartova, Jirina; Ulcova-Gallova, Zdena; Mrklas, Lubor; and Stejskal, Vera D. Sensitization to Inorganic Mercury Could Be a Risk Factor for Infertility. *Neuroendocrinol Lett* 2005; 26(4); 277-282.

Prochazkova, Jarmila; Sterzl, Ivan; Kucerova, Hana; Bartova, Jirina; and Stejskal, Vera D. The Beneficial Effect of Amalgam Replacement on Health in Patients with Autoimmunity. Neuroendocrinol Lett 2004; 25(3); 211-218.

Tibbling, L.; Thuomas, K.; Lenkei, R.; and Stejskal, V. Immunological and Brain MRI Changes in Patients with Suspected Metal Intoxication. International Journal of Occupational Medicine and Toxicology, Vol. 4, No. 2, 1995, pp. 285-294.

U.S. Environmental Protection Agency. Last updated Aug. 6, 2009. Mercury: Consumer and Commercial Products. www.epa.gov/mercury/consumer.htm. Last accessed Sept. 6, 2009.

U.S. Environmental Protection Agency. Last updated Aug. 3, 2009. Mercury: EPA's Roadmap for Mercury, Executive Summary. www.epa.gov/mercury/executivesummary.htm. Last accessed Sept. 6, 2009.

U.S. Environmental Protection Agency. Last updated 02/07/2012. Mercury: Health Effects. www.epa.gov/mercury/effects.htm. Last accessed Jan. 13, 2013.

U.S. Environmental Protection Agency. Last updated 08/06/2009. Mercury: Laws and Regulations. www.epa.gov/mercury/regs.htm. Last accessed Sept. 6, 2009.

U.S. Environmental Protection Agency. Last updated March 23, 2009. Mercury: State Legislation and Regulations. www.epa.gov/osw/hazard/tsd/mercury/laws.htm. Last accessed Sept. 6, 2009.

U.S. Environmental Protection Agency. July 2005. Mercury-Containing Equipment Classified as Universal Waste. EPA530-F-05-010. www.epa/gov/osw. Last accessed March 22, 2009.

U.S. Environmental Protection Agency. Last updated 11/06/2007. Technology Transfer Network Air Toxics Web Site Mercury Compounds. www.epa.gov/ttnatw01/hlthef/mercury.html. Last accessed Jan. 13, 2013.

U.S. Food and Drug Administration. Consumer Updates: Mercury Poisoning Linked to Skin Products. www.fda.gov/ForConsumers/ConsumerUpdates/ucm294849.htm#1. Last updated Aug. 9, 2012. Last accessed January 13, 2013.

U.S. Food and Drug Administration. July 28, 2009. *FINAL RULE: Dental Devices: Classification of Dental Amalgam, Reclassification of Dental Mercury,* Designation of Special Controls for Dental Amalgam, Mercury, and Amalgam Alloy. 21 CFR Part 872 [Docket No. FDA-2008-N-0163] (formerly Docket No. 2001N-0067). www.fda.gov. Last accessed Sept. 1, 2009.

U.S. Food and Drug Administration. *Medical Devices: About Dental Amalgam Fillings.* www.fda.gov/MedicalDevices/ProductsandMedicalProcedures/DentalProducts/DentalAmalgam/ucm171094.htm. Last updated Aug. 11, 2009. Last accessed Jan. 13, 2013.

U.S. Food and Drug Administration, Department of Health and Human Services. 21 CFR Part 872. *Dental Devices: Classification of Dental*

Amalgam, Reclassification of Dental Mercury, Designation of Special Controls for Dental Amalgam, Mercury, and Amalgam Alloy.

Windham, Bernie (ed). *Dental Amalgam Fillings* Page. www.flcv.com. Last accessed March 22, 2009.

Windham, Bernard (ed). *Mercury Exposure Levels from Amalgam Dental Fillings; Documentation of Mechanisms by which Mercury Causes Over 40 Chronic Health Conditions; Results of Replacement of Amalgam Fillings; and Occupational Effects on Dental Staff.* Tallahassee, FL ,323 11 850-878-9024. www.fda.gov. Last accessed Jan. 13, 2013.

Ziff, Sam, and Ziff, Michael F. *Dentistry Without Mercury.* 1995 ed. Bio-Probe Inc. Orlando, FL.

- Chapter 8 -
The Dangers of Root Canal-Treated Teeth

Cancer-Free Newsletter. Dec. 8, 2005. Dr. Rau's *Experience with Cancer and Root Canals.* www.beating-cancer-gently.com/nl89.html. Last accessed Jan. 4, 2013.

Dowling, Bob. July 14, 2010. *Curing Breast Cancer with Dr. Bob Dowling.* oneradionetwork.com. Last accessed Jan. 7, 2013. Podcast.

Dowling, Bob. May 12, 2011. *Curing Cancer: The Politics of Health.* The Morning Show with Patrick Timpone. oneradionetwork.com. Last accessed Jan. 7, 2013. Radio interview.

Dowling, Bob. Dec. 6, 2008. *The Teeth and Jawbone - Certain Link to Cancer.* oneradionetwork.com. Last accessed Jan. 7, 2013. Podcast.

Goldman, Michael C. *Root Canal Treatment Choices* www.mgoldmandds. com/rctchoices.htm. Last accessed Jan. 4, 2013.

Issels, Josef. Cancer: *A Second Opinion: A Look at Understanding, Controlling, and Curing Cancer.* London: Hodder and Stoughton, 1975. Print.

Kulacz, Robert and Levy, Thomas E. (2014). *The Toxic Tooth, How a root canal could be making you sick.* MedFox Publishing, LLC.

Lee, Laura. *Cavitations & Root Canals. Interview with George Meinig, D.D.S and Dr. M. LaMarche.* A Talk Show hosted by Laura Lee. First aired May 20, 1995. http://www.tldp.com/issue/157-8/157rootc.htm. Last accessed Dec. 18, 2012.

Meinig, George E. (1994). *Root Canal Cover-Up* (Second Edition). http://books.google.com/books/about/Root_Canal_Cover_ Up.html?id=LxhqAAAAMAAJ Bion Publishing.

Mercola, Joseph. *Root Canals Pose Health Threat.* Interview with George Meinig, D.D.S. http://www.mercola.com/article/dental/rootcanal/root_ canals.htm Last accessed June 16, 2009.

Price, Weston A., D.D.S. Nutrition and Physical Degeneration. Price-Pottenger Nutrition Foundation, La Mesa, CA, 1945, 1979.

Rau, Thomas, Dr., medical director, Paracelsus Clinic in Switzerland. The Morning Show with Patrick Timpone. June 27, 2011. http://oneradionetwork.com/health/dr-thomas-rau-holistic-physician-june-27-2011/ Last accessed Jan. 7, 2013. Radio interview.

- Chapter 9 -
Why and How Should Extracted Teeth be Replaced?

Clifford, Walter J. Personal Communications, June 13, 2012.

Clifford, Walter J. Personal Communications, Sept. 29, 2009.

Chaturvedi, T.P. An Overview of the Corrosion Aspect of Dental Implants (Titanium And Its Alloys). Indian Journal of Dental Research, 20(1), 2009. Pp 91-98.

Depprich, R.; Zipprich, H.; Ommerborn, M.; Naujoks, C.; Wiesmann, H.P.; Kiattavorncharoen, S.; Lauer, H.C.; Meyer, U.; Kubler, N.R.; and Handschel J. Osseointegration of Zirconia Implants Compared With Titanium: An In Vivo Study. Head & Face Medicine 2008, 4:30.

Dorner, T.; Haas, J.; Loddenkemper, C.; von Baehr, V.; and Salama, A. Implant-Related Inflammatory Arthritis. Nature Clinical Practice Rheumatology, January 2006, Vol. 2, No. 1, pp. 53-56.

Hentges, Steven G. Bisphenol-A in Dental Composites. Original article at http://www.bisphenol-a.org/human/dental.html. Reproduced in 2007 by IAOMT at www.iaomt.org. Last accessed Sept. 8, 2009.

Hyams B.L. and Ballon H.C. Dissimilar Metals in the Mouth as a Possible Cause of Otherwise Unexplainable Symptoms. Can. M. J. 29: 488, 1932.

Ionescu, J.G.; Novotny, J; Stejskal, V.D.; Latsch, A.; Blaurock-Busch, E.; Eisenmann-Klein, M. Increased levels of Transition Metals in Breast Cancer Tissue. Neuro Endocrinol Lett. 2006; 27(Suppl1): 36-39.

Lambrich, M.; Iglhaut, G. Comparison of the Survival Rates for Zirconia and Titanium Implants. JDI Journal of Dental Implantology. Vol. 24, No. 3, 2008, pp. 182-191.

Magnusson, B.; Bergman, M.; Bergman, B.; Sörenmark, R. Nickel Allergy and Nickel-Containing Dental Alloys. Scand J Dent Res. 1982 Apr; 90(2): 163-7.

McGuff, H.S.; Heim-Hall, J.; Holsinger, C.F.; Jones. A.A.; O'Dell, D.S.; Hafemeister, AC. Maxillary Osteosarcoma Associated with a Dental Implant: Report of a Case and Review of the Literature Regarding Implant-Related Sarcomas. JADA, Vol. 139. August 2008. Pp. 1052-1059.

Muller, K; Valentine-Thon, E. Hypersensitivity to Titanium: Clinical and Laboratory Evidence. Neuroendocrinol Lett 2006; 27(Suppl 1):31-35.

Muris, J.; Feilzer, A.J. Microanalysis of Metals in Dental Restorations as Part of a Diagnostic Approach in Metal Allergies. *Neuro Endocrinol Lett.* 2006; 27(Suppl1): 49-52.

Ndebele, Kenneth; Tchounwou, Paul B.; and McMurray, Robert W. Effects of Xenoestrogens on T Lymphocytes: Modulation of bcl-2, p53, and Apoptosis. *Int. J. Mol. Sci.* 2003, 4, 45-61.

Oliva, J.; Oliva, X.; Oliva, J.D. *One-year Follow-Up of First Consecutive 100 Zirconia Dental Implants in Humans: A Comparison of 2 Different Rough Surfaces.*

Schriever, W.; Diamond, L.E. Electromotive Forces and Electric Currents Cause by Metallic Dental Fillings. *Journal of Dental Research,* Apr 1952; vol. 31: pp. 205-229

ScienceDaily. 04/22/2008. *Chemical in Plastic Bottles Raises Some Concern, According to New Report.* Available at www.sciencedaily.com. Last accessed Sept. 8, 2009.

Stejskal, V.D.M.; Cederbrant, K.; Lindvall, A.; Forsbeck, M. MELISA - An In-Vitro Tool for the Study of Metal Allergy. *Toxic in Vitro* Vol. 8, No. 5, pp. 991-1000, 1994. Printed in Great Britain.

Stejskal, V.D.M.; Danersund, A.; Lindvall, A.; Hudecek, R.; Nordman, V.; Yaqob, A.; Mayer, W.; Bieger, W.; and Lindh, U. Metal-Specific Lymphocytes: Biomarkers of Sensitivity in Man. *Neuro Endocrinol Lett* 1999; 20:289-298.

Stejskal, V.D.; Hudecek, R.; Stejskal, J.; Sterzl, I. Diagnosis and Treatment of Metal-Induced Side Effects. *Neuro Endocrinol Lett* 2006; 27 (Suppl 1): 7-16.

Stejskal, J.; Stejskal, V.D.M. The Role of Metals in Autoimmunity and the Link to Neuroendocrinology. *Neuro Endocrinol Lett* 1999; 20:351-364.

Sterzl, I.; Prochazkova, J.; Hrda, P.; Bartova, J.; Matucha, P.; Stejskal, V.D.M. Mercury and Nickel Allergy: Risk Factors in Fatigue and Autoimmunity. *Neuro Endocrinol Lett* 1999; 20:221-228.

Valentine-Thon, E.; Muller, K.; Guzzi, G.; Kreisel, S.; Ohnsorge, P.; and Sandkamp M. LTT-MELISA® Is Clinically Relevant for Detecting and Monitoring Metal Sensitivity. *Neuro Endocrinol Lett* 2006; 27(Suppl 1):17-24.

- Chapter 10 & 11 -
Getting Your Nutrition Right &
Eating in Harmony with Your Metabolism

Fallon, Sally. July 2004. *The Pioneering Research of Dr. Weston A. Price: The Whole, Natural Food Diet.* www.nourishingwisdom.com. Last accessed March 7, 2009.

Marlowe, Jim: Consultation and Nutritional Advice, 2009-2012.

Price-Pottenger Nutrition Foundation. *What Is The Price-Pottenger Nutrition Foundation?* www.ppnf.org Last accessed March 7, 2009.

The Weston A. Price Foundation. Weston A. Price, DDS. http://westonaprice. org Last accessed March 7, 2009.

- Chapter 12 -
Fluoride is Not Your Friend

American Dental Association (ADA). *American Dental Association Supports Fluoridation.* Available at http://www.ada.org/2092.aspx. Page Updated Nov. 22, 2002. Last accessed Jan. 13, 2013.

American Dental Association (ADA) (2005). *Fluoridation Facts.* Available at http://www.ada.org/sections/newsAndEvents/pdfs/fluoridation_facts.pdf (last accessed Dec. 18, 2012).

Bassin, E.B.; Wypij, D.; Davis, R.B.; and Mitleman, M.A. (May 2006). Age-Specific Fluoride Exposure in Drinking Water and Osteosarcoma (United States). *Cancer Causes Control.* 2006 May; 17(4):481-2.

Bernays, Edward L. 1923. *Crystallizing Public Opinion.* New York: Liveright Publishing Corp.

Bernays, Edward L. 1928. *Propaganda.* New York: H. Liveright.

Blaylock, R. (2006). http://www.cdc.gov/FLUORIDATION/fact_sheets/osteo-sarcoma.htm Page last modified Sept. 17, 2007; last accessed June 12, 2009.

Centers for Disease Control and Prevention. *Community Water Fluoridation.* Available at http://www.cdc.gov/fluoridation/. Page last updated: Oct. 31, 2012. Last accessed Jan. 13, 2013.

Centers for Disease Control and Prevention. *Engineering and Administrative Recommendations for Water Fluoridation,* 1995. MMWR Sept. 29, 1995; 44 (No. RR-13); 1-40.

Centers for Disease Control and Prevention (2008). *Other Fluoride Products.* http://www.cdc.gov/fluoridation/other.htm. (Date last reviewed: Oct. 8, 2008. Date last modified: Aug. 9, 2007. Last accessed June 12, 2009).

Centers for Disease Control and Prevention. *Recommendations for Using Fluoride to Prevent and Control Dental Caries in the United States.* MMWR Aug. 17, 2001; 50 (No. RR-14); 1-42.

Chemical Commodities Agency. *MSDS: Sodium Silicofluoride, Technical.* 01/01/1987. http://hazard.com/msds. Last accessed March 22, 2009.

Chemtech Industries Inc. MSDS: *Sodium Fluoride, Powder.* 03/29/1988. http://hazard.com/msds. Last accessed March 22, 2009.

Chemtech Industries Inc. *MSDS: Sodium Silicofluoride.* 01/01/1987. http://hazard.com/msds. Last accessed March 22, 2009.

Chol, A.L.; Sun, G.; Zhang, Y.; Grandjean, P. Developmental Fluoride Neurotoxicity: A Systematic Review and Meta-Analysis. *Environ Health*

Perspect 120:1362-1368 (2012). http://dx.doi.org/10.1289/ehp.1104912 [Online 20 July 2012]

Collaborative on Health and the Environment's Learning and Developmental Disabilities Initiative (2008). Scientific Consensus Statement on Environmental Agents Associated with Neurodevelopmental Disorders. http://www.iceh.org/pdfs/LDDI/LDDIStatement.pdf Last accessed May 8, 2009.

Connett M. *The Phosphate Fertilizer Industry: An Environmental Overview.* Fluoride Action Network. May 2003. Available at http://www.fluoridealert. org/articles/phosphate01/. Last accessed Jan. 13, 2013.

Connett, P. (updated Sept. 2012). *50 Reasons to Oppose Fluoridation.* Available at http://www.fluoridealert.org/articles/50-reasons/ Last accessed Dec. 18, 2012.

Connett, P; Beck, J.; Micklem, H.S. 2010. *The Case Against Fluoride: How Hazardous Waste Ended Up in Our Drinking Water and the Bad Science and Powerful Politics that Keep It There.* Chelsea Green Publishing Company, White River Junction, Vermont.

Erdal, S. and Buchanan, S.N. (Jan. 2005). A Quantitative Look at Fluorosis, Fluoride Exposure, and Intake in Children Using a Health-Risk Assessment Approach. *Environ Health Perspect.* 2005 January; 113(1): 111-117. (Published online 2004 Sept. 14. doi: 10.1289/ehp.7077).

Fisher Scientific. *MSDS: Sodium Fluoride.* MSDS Creation Date: 7/07/1999. Revision #6 Date: 2/15/2008. http://fscimage.fishersci.com/msds/21230. htm. Last accessed March 22, 2009.

Fluoride Action Network. *Communities Which Have Rejected Fluoridation Since 1990.* Available at http://www.fluoridealert.org/communities.htm Last accessed March 15, 2009.

Gosselin R.E.; Smith, R.P.; Hodge, H.C.; Braddock, J.E. *Clinical Toxicology of Commercial Products* (5th ed). Williams & Wilkins, 1984.

Hankel-Khan, Gerda. Sept. 16, 1999. Letter from Gerda Hankel-Khan, Embassy of the Federal Republic of Germany, to A.R. Smith, Nr Stroke on Trent, Staffs ST9 9JP. www.fluoridealert.org/Germany.jpeg. Last accessed March 31, 2009.

Hanmer, Rebecca. March 30, 1983. Letter from Rebecca Hanmer, deputy assistant administrator for water, to Leslie A. Russell, D.M.D. http://www. fluoridealert.org/uploads/hanmer1983.pdf. Last accessed Jan. 13, 2013.

Hiisvirta, Leena. Jan. 12, 1996. Letter from Leena Hiisvirta, chief engineer, Helsinki, Finland, to Elroy Belbeck, president, Fluoride-Free Association, Owen Sound, ON, Canada. www.fluoridealert.org/finland.jpeg. Last accessed March 31, 2009.

International Academy of Oral Medicine and Toxicology (January 2003). *Policy Position on Ingested Fluoride and Fluoridation.* Posted Sept. 22, 2006. Last accessed Dec. 18, 2012, at http://iaomt.guiadmin.com/wp-content/uploads/article_IAOMT-Fluoridation-Position.pdf

J.T. Baker Chemical Co. *MSDS: Sodium Fluoride.* Oct. 15, 1987. http://hazard. com/msds. Last accessed March 22, 2009.

Mallinckrodt Baker, Inc. *MSDS: Sodium Fluoride.* MSDS Number S3722. 11/26/2007. www.jtbaker.com. Last accessed March 22, 2009.

National Research Council (2006). *Fluoride in Drinking Water: A Scientific Review of EPA's Standards.* Available from the National Academies Press, 500 Fifth Street, NW, Washington, D.C. 20001; (800) 624-6242; www.nap. edu.

National Research Council (March 2006). *Report in Brief: Fluoride in Drinking Water: A Scientific Review of EPA's Standards.* National Academy of Sciences. http://dels.nas.edu/dels/rpt_briefs/fluoride_brief_final.pdf (last accessed May 8, 2009).

"Propaganda." Oxford English Dictionary Online. Oxford University Press. n.d. Web. Jan. 10, 2013.

Ries, Jean-Marie. May 3, 2000. Letter from Jean-Marie Ries, head of the Water Department, Luxembourg, to Eugene Albright, North Versailles, PA, U.S.A. www.fluoridealert.org/luxembourg.jpeg. Last accessed March 31, 2009.

Ripa, Louis W. (Winter 1993). A Half-Century of Community Water Fluoridation in the United States: Review and Commentary. *J Public Health Dent* 1993; 53(1): 17-44.

Schuld, Andreas; Small, Wendy. *Another Fluoride Drug Bites the Dust.* http:// articles.mercola.com/sites/articles/archive/2001/08/18/fluoride-drugs. aspx Aug. 18, 2001.

The National Academies (March 2006). *Fluoride in Drinking Water: A Scientific Review of EPA's Standards.* National Academies Press, Washington, D.C.

UNICEF (December 1999). A Future Global Agenda for Children: The Links with Sanitation, Hygiene, Water and Environment. *WATERfront*: Issue 13: December 1999. http://www.unicef.org/wash/files/wf13e.pdf

U.S. Food and Drug Administration (July 2005). *FDA Announces Withdrawal Fenfluramine and Dexfenfluramine (Fen-Phen).* http://www.fda.gov/Drugs/DrugSafety/ PostmarketDrugSafetyInformationforPatientsandProviders/ucm179871. htm Date created: Sept. 15, 1997; Last update: July 7, 2005. Last accessed: March 17, 2009.

U.S. Department of Agriculture. *USDA National Fluoride Database of Selected Beverages and Foods.* October 2004. Available at http://www/ nal/usda/gov/fnic/foodcomp Last accessed March 29, 2009

World Health Organization 2004. *Fluoride in Drinking Water, Background Document for Development of WHO Guidelines for Drinking Water Quality.* Last accessed March 14, 2009.

World Health Organization. 2006. *Fluoride in Drinking Water.* IWA Publishing, Alliance House, 12 Caxton Street, London SW1H 0QS, UK. Last accessed

May 8, 2009. http://www.who.int/water_sanitation_health/publications/flu-oride_drinking_water_full.pdf

World Health Organization. *WHO Oral Health Country/Area Profile Programme.* Department of Noncommunicable Diseases Surveillance/ Oral Health. WHO Collaborating Centre, Malmö University, Sweden.

O ―――――

oil pulling *205, 206, 207, 208, 209*

olive oil *206*

onlay *63, 64*

oral hygiene *39, 139, 140, 201, 208*

OSHA - Occupational Safety and
    Health Administration *72*

osteomyelitis *223*

osteonecrosis *223*

Osteonecrosis *223*

osteopath *229, 243*

osteopathic *7, 225, 226, 228, 229, 230, 231, 232*

oxygen *102, 138, 211, 212, 213, 215,
    221, 222, 227, 231, 232*

ozonated gas *213*

ozonated water *214, 215*

P ―――――

partial *64, 94, 131, 132, 133, 135*

Pathogens, Dental/Oral

perceptual abilities *228*

periodontal disease *39, 50, 88, 89,
    105, 174, 213, 214, 227*

periodontitis *46, 57, 82, 86, 87, 89, 105, 136*

phosphate fertilizer industry *194*

pineal gland *199*

plaque *91, 205, 227, 231*

poison *46, 50, 75, 83*

polish *208*

porcelain *66, 67, 133, 134, 135*

Price, Weston *107, 108, 109, 110, 111, 112, 113,
    114, 117, 118, 119, 122, 124, 125, 127, 146,
    147, 148, 149, 150, 151, 200, 250, 251, 252*

Made in the USA
Monee, IL
02 May 2025

16757941R00148